THIS BOOK

BELONGS TO

....

....

Author's Afterthoughts

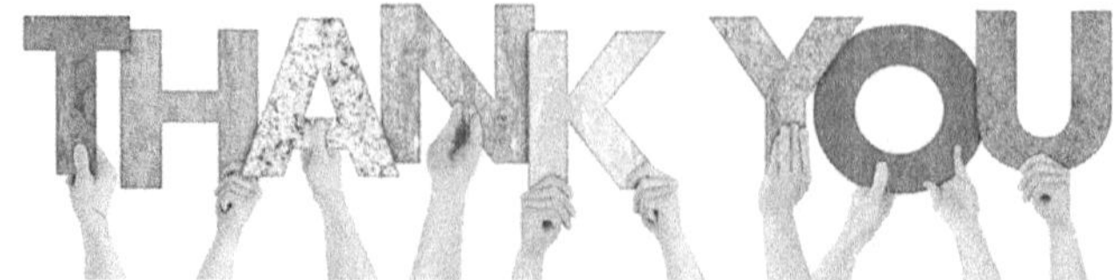

With so many books out there to choose from, I want to thank you for choosing this one and taking precious time out of your life to buy and read my work. Readers like you are the reason I take such passion in creating these books.

It is with gratitude and humility that I express how honored I am to become a part of your life and I hope that you take the same pleasure in reading this book as I did in writing it.

Can I ask one small favour? I ask that you write an honest and open review on Amazon of what you thought of the book. This will help other readers make an informed choice on whether to buy this book.

My sincerest thanks.

Table of Contents

INTRODUCTION

The key advantages of autophagy tend to come in the form of the concepts of anti-aging. Indeed, Petre says it is best known as the manner in which the body turns the clock back and produces younger cells. Scintits

Scientists point out that autophagy is enhanced when our cells are stressed, to support us, which helps to boost the lifespan.

In addition, registered dietitian, Scott Keatley, RD, CDN, says autophagy keeps the body working in times of malnutrition by breaking down biological material and reusing it for essential processes.

"Of course, it requires energy and can not continue indefinitely, but it allows us more time to find nourishment" At the cellular level, Petre says that the advantages of autophagy include: eliminating toxic proteins from cells that are due to neurodegenerative diseases, such as Parkinson's and Alzheimer's disease, recycling residual proteins that provide energy and building blocks for cells that are still capable of growing.

"Autophagy decreases as we age, and this means cells that can no longer function or do harm will spread, which is the MO of cancer cells,".

Although all cancers originate from some kind of defective cells, Petre says the body should recognize those cells and remove them, sometimes using autophagic processes. This is why some researchers are looking into the possibility this autophagy can reduce cancer risk.

Although there is no conclusive evidence to back this up, Petre says some reports indicate that autophagy can kill many cancer cells.

"This is how the body protects heroes against cancer," she says. "Recognizing and repairing what went wrong and activating the repair mechanism helps to minimize the risk of cancer." Researchers hope new research will lead to findings that will help them approach autophagy as a cancer therapy.

Note that autophagy simply means "self-eating." Therefore it makes sense for autophagy to be caused by intermittent fasting and ketogenic diets.

"Fasting is the most powerful form of inducing autophagy," Petre states.

"Ketosis, a diet high in fat and low in carbohydrates, offers the same advantages of fasting without fasting as a way to cause the same beneficial changes in metabolism," she said. "By not loading the body with an external load, it gives the body a break to concentrate on its own health and repair." In the keto diet, you get about 75% of your daily calories from fat, and about 5% to 10% of your calories from the carbohydrates.

This change in sources of calories is causing the body to move its metabolic pathways. Instead of the glucose that is extracted from carbohydrates it will continue using fat for fuel.

Your body will begin to produce ketone bodies which have several protective effects in response to this restriction. Khorana says studies indicate that ketosis, which has neuroprotective functions, may also cause starvation-induced autophagy.

"Both diets show low levels of glucose and are related to low levels of insulin and high levels of glucagon," Petre says. And the degree of the glucagon is that which initiates autophagy.

"When the body, by fasting or ketosis, is low in sugar it brings the positive stress that wakes up the mode of survival repair," she adds.

Exercise is one non-diet region which may also play a part in inducing autophagy. Physical exercise can induce autophagy in organs which are part of the processes of metabolic control.

This may include tissue from the lungs, liver, pancreas and adipose.

As researchers perform more studies on the effect it has on our health, the bottom line Autophagy will continue to get publicity.

Right now, nutritional and wellness experts are referring to the fact that we still have a lot to know about autophagy and how to better promote it.

But if you want to try to induce autophagy in your body, she advises that you start by incorporating fasting and daily exercise to your routine.

Nevertheless, if you are taking any medicine, are pregnant, breastfeeding, or would like to become pregnant, or have a medical illness, such as heart disease or diabetes, you need to contact your doctor.

I caution that if you fall into any of the above categories, you are not encouraged to fast.

LET'S GET INTO MORE DETAILS!!!

CHAPTER 1: AUTOPHAGY AND AGING?

What defines autophagy? The Greek term derives from auto (self) and phagein (eat). Therefore the term basically means eating yourself. Essentially, this is the body's process to get rid of all the broken down, old cell machinery (organels, proteins, and cell membranes) because there is not enough capacity to support it any longer. The degradation and recycling of cellular components is controlled, orderly process.

There is a related, better known mechanism also known as programmed cell death called apoptosis. Cells are programmed to die after a certain number of divisions. Although this can at first sound like macabre, remember that this phase is important to preserving good health. Suppose you possess a car, for example. You love the car. You've had big experiences in it. You just enjoy riding it.

Yet it starts looking sort of beat-up after a few years. It doesn't look so amazing, after a few more. The vehicle costs you thousands of dollars for repairs each year. Every rest of the time, it breaks down. Is it easier to keep that around because it's just a hunk of junk? Of course not. Yeah, you're getting rid of it and buying a fancy new car.

The same is true in the body. Cells are getting old, and junky. It's easier to get them programmed to die when their useful lives are finished. It really sounds cruel but it's life. This is the apoptosis cycle, where cells are pre-destined to die after some time. This is like leasing an vehicle. You get rid of the car after a certain amount of time, whether it is still going or not. Then you buy yourself a new car. You should not think about breaking it down at the worst possible moment.

On a subcellular stage too, the same process happens. You don't have to replace the whole car, necessarily. You just have to remove the battery occasionally, chuck the old one out and get a new one. This happens in the cells, too. Instead of destroying the entire cell (apoptosis) you just want to destroy certain pieces of the cell. This is the autophagy cycle, where subcellular organelles are killed and new ones are created to replace them. You should extract old membranes, organelles, and other cellular waste. It is achieved by sending it to the lysosome that is a specialized organelle that includes protein degrading enzymes.

Autophagy was first described in 1962, when researchers observed an increase in the number of lysosomes(the part of the cell that destroys junk) in rat liver cells after infusing glucagon. The word autophagy was coined by Nobel laureate scientist Christian de Duve. Damaged subcellular sections and unused proteins are marked for destruction and then sent to the lysosomes for completion of the work.

One of the main autophagy regulators is a kinase known as rapamycin (mTOR) mammalian target. It suppresses autophagy when mTOR is activated, and encourages it when dormant.

Deprivation of nutrients is the main activator of autophagy. Recall that insulin is kind of the opposite hormone to glucagon. It's like the game that we played as youngsters-' opposite day.' If insulin goes up, then glucagon will go down. If insulin goes down, then glucagon will go up. The sugar goes up when we chew, and the glucagon goes down. If we don't eat (fast) insulin will go down, and glucagon will go up. The glucagon increase activates the autophagy cycle.

Fasting (raises glucagon) potentially gives the biggest known boost to autophagy.

Fasting is also much more effective than merely inducing autophagy. They're doing two good things. We're cleaning out all our old, junky proteins and cellular pieces by inducing autophagy. Simultaneously, fasting also activates growth hormone, which tells our body to start creating some new snazzy body parts. We are also giving the entire renovation to our bodies.

You need to get rid of the old things before you can bring new things in. Dream about getting your kitchen renovated. If you have old lime green cabinets sitting around in the 1970s era, you need to trash them before you bring any new ones in. Therefore, the destruction process (removal) is just as critical as the production process. If you were simply trying to bring the old cabinets in without taking them out, it wouldn't look so bright. So fasting can reverse the aging process in some ways, by getting rid of old cellular junk and replacing it with new pieces.

Autophagy is a process which has strong regulations. That would be harmful if it runs amok out of reach, so it must be carefully managed. Total loss of amino acids in mammalian cells is a strong signal for autophagy but more variable is the position of individual amino acids. The levels of amino acid in the plasma differ just a little, though. Signals of amino acids and growth factor / insulin signals are thought to converge on the mTOR pathway-also called the nutrient signaling master regulator.

Therefore, during autophagy, components of old cells are broken down into the amino acid portion (the protein building block). That happens to amino acids like this? The amino acid levels begin to increase in the early stages of starvation. Those amino acids derived from autophagy are thought to be provided for gluconeogenesis to the liver. They may also be broken down into glucose through the cycle of tricarboxylic acid (TCA). The third potential fate of amino acids will be introduced into new proteins.

Two major disorders–Alzheimer's Disease (AD) and cancer–will see the effects of storing old junky proteins all over the place. Alzheimer's disease involves the accumulation of defective protein-namely amyloid beta or Tau protein that gums the brain structure upwards. While we do not yet have proof of clinical trials for this, it would make sense that a mechanism like autophagy that has the potential to clean out old protein could prevent AD from forming.

Who disables autophagy? Water. Glucose, insulin (or glucagon decreased), and proteins all switching this self-cleaning cycle off. And it doesn't need a number. Only a small amount of amino acid (leucine) could halt cold autophagy. This cycle of autophagy is also peculiar to fasting-something that is not present in normal caloric restriction or diet.

There is of course a balance here. You get sick both because of too much autophagy and too little. Which brings us back to life's natural cycle-fast and festive. Not smooth diet. This helps the growth of cells during feeding, and cellular cleaning during fasting-balance. Life is all about equilibrium.

Let's continue by exploring what aging is. Everyone knows instinctively what it means to age, but science takes a specific description to solve any issue successfully. We can see ageing in a variety of ways.

Second, because of a shift of appearance, ageing is also apparent. Gray hair, wrinkled skin and age shows other superficial changes. These physical changes indicate underlying physiological changes, such as decreased development of pigments in hair follicles and decreased elasticity in skin. Cosmetic surgery alters appearance but not the physiology that underlies it.

Third, we can see aging as a functional loss. Over time, in a cycle mostly dictated by age, women have rising fertility before ovulation finally stops during menopause altogether. Bones are weaker, through the likelihood of breaks such as hip fractures, issues that we seldom see in children. Muscles are also getting smaller, which explains why champion athletes are still young.

Third, with age, response to hormones decreases at the cellular and molecular levels. For example, if your cells no longer respond to certain hormones, high insulin (a fat-and glucose-storing hormone) or thyroid hormone levels do not help you much. Mitochondria, the essential cellular components that produce energy and are widely referred to as the "cell's engine," are less efficient and less capable of generating energy. Ageing body's decreasing productivity results in higher rates of disease and illness.

Increasing age raises the risk of sickness and death exponentially. For example, heart attacks are practically absent in children but common in older people. Aging is not a disease itself but it raises the risk of contracting diseases, making it the best target for chronic diseases to avoid or reverse. Age is a river of historical years-permanent and flowing of one direction. Yet aging is not the case, in physiological years. Several factors contribute to aging and disease, and in this book, we find mainly the aspects affected by diet.

EVOLUTION DOESN'T CARE WHETHER YOU AGE

Why are organisms aging at all despite the overall functional decline? In short, aging is damage accumulation. Young animals, including humans, have a strong ability to repair daily damage, such as when kids scratch their knees. Survival of species depends on the ability to repair this damage: in healing wounds or broken bones for example. Over age, this capacity to heal damage in all respects diminishes— whether to combat infections, clear lungs, or destroy cancer cells. The decline, however, is not a natural, foregone conclusion. Most of the speed and severity of the aging process is dictated by diet and lifestyle. Long-lived, healthy populations worldwide that consume few processed foods give us the prospect of slowing down the aging cycle.

Ancient Greek father of modern medicine, Hippocrates long ago accepted diet as the foundation of health and longevity. Famine is one of the Apocalypse's Four Horsemen but the modern issues of obesity, insulin resistance, and diabetes are just as lethal. In both cases, the foods we consume play a significant role in the production or prevention of both of these issues.

One essential mechanism for damage-repair is called autophagy. (The fact that Yoshinori Ohsumi was awarded the 2016 Nobel Prize in Medicine for his "discoveries of autophagy processes" underlines how important this process is.) In autophagy, cellular components called organelles are broken down and replaced periodically as part of a large quality control system. Just like a car requires daily oil, filters, and belts replacement, a cell has to periodically change its organelles to maintain normal function. As cellular organelles reach their expiration dates, the body ensures the removal and replacement of old organelles with new ones so that no residual damage impedes work. One of the main findings of the last quarter century is that the food we consume greatly affects these procedures for damage control.

You would think our damage control responses will be mastered by evolution, allowing us to live for ever. But evolution doesn't matter whether you're dying or just alive. It ensures the species, not the human, will survive. When you have offsprings, and if you don't, your genes will survive, and there's no natural selection to longer-lived species. The rationale is behind the aging theory known as antagonistic pleiotropy. The theory, given its name, is fairly basic.

Natural selection evolution functions at gene level, rather than for individual species. We all bear and pass forth thousands of different genes to our babies. Genes that are best suited to the environment of the individual survive better and allow the individual to produce more offspring. Those beneficial genes are becoming more common in the population over time. Age plays a major role in deciding the impact a gene has on the population.

A gene that is lethal at the age of 10 (before a person has children) is easily removed from the population because it cannot be passed on by the person carrying the gene. A gene that is lethal at age 30 can still be removed (although more slowly), as more children are available to people without that gene. A gene that is lethal at 70 years of age may never be removed because the gene may have passed into the next generation long before its deadly effects manifest.

Antagonistic pleiotropy indicates that, at various periods of life, genes have different effects. For example, a gene which increases growth and fertility but also increases cancer risk in old age means more children but a shorter life span. This gene will still spread in a given population, since evolution prefers gene survival, not a human life's longevity. One gene can have two separate, unrelated effects (pleiotropy), which are clearly at odds with each other (antagonistic). Gene survival is often given priority over human longevity.

This particular gene mentioned codes for a protein known as the growth factor 1 (IGF-1) similar to insulin. High levels of IGF-1 promote growth, allowing organisms to grow larger, multiply faster, and have better weather wounds. That is a huge advantage to survive in competition to have kids. High IGF-1 leads to cancer, heart disease, and early death in old age, however, and by that time, the gene has already passed into the next generation. When growth / reproduction faces longevity, evolution supports reproduction and high rates of IGF-1. That is the fundamental and natural balance between longevity and development.

Seen in this sense, fighting the ravages of aging is a war against nature itself. Although the degree and speed are variable, ageing is absolutely normal. Living and eating in perfect harmony with nature does not prevent ageing. Nature and evolution will not "look out" for your longevity; the only concern is the survival of your genes. In a way, to slow down or avoid aging, we have to look beyond nature.

EVOLUTIONARILY CONSERVED MECHANISMS

Simple one-celled organisms, or prokaryotes, such as bacteria, are the earliest life forms on earth and exist today. Eukaryotes, more complex but still monocellular organisms, first emerged around 1.5 billion years later. The multicellular life-forms called metazoans originated from those modest beginnings. All the animal cells are eukaryotic cells, even in humans. They bear a similarity to each other, since they share a similar heritage. Most molecular processes (genes, proteins, and so on) and biochemical pathways are conserved for more complex organisms during evolution.

Human beings associate with chimpanzees with around 98.8 per cent of our chromosomes. This genetic variation of 1.2 per cent is adequate to compensate for the variations between the two species. It may be even more shocking to discover that species have no genes in common, as far apart as yeast and humans. At least 20 per cent of human genes that play a role in causing disease have yeast counterparts. Once scientists spliced over 400 different human genes into the Saccharomyces cerevisiae yeast, they found that the genes of the yeast were functionally replaced by a full 47 per cent.

We find even bigger parallels with more complex species, such as the mouse. Among the more than 4,000 genes analyzed, less than 10 were found to vary between mice and humans. Of all protein-coding genes— excluding the so-called "junk" DNA— mice and human genes are similar in 85 per cent. Mice and humans are genetically very close.

Many aging-related genes are retained in the population, enabling scientists to research yeast and mice to learn essential human biology lessons. Many of the studies discussed in this book include species as diverse as yeast, rodents, and rhesus monkeys and differ in the degree to which they are analogous to humans. Not every outcome applies to humans, but in most cases the findings are similar enough to allow you to learn a lot from them about ageing. Though human studies are ideal, these do not occur in many situations, which causes us to rely on animal studies.

THEORIES OF AGING

The following paragraphs describe the concepts of different ageing theories and our judgment on each's plausibility.

DISPOSABLE SOMA THEORY

The disposable soma theory of aging, initially proposed by Professor Thomas Kirkwood at the University of Newcastle, holds that species have a finite amount of energy that can be used either in body maintenance and repair (soma) or in reproduction. There is a trade-off like antagonistic pleiotropy: If you reserve energy for maintenance and repair, you have less resources available for reproduction. Since evolution directs more energy towards reproduction, which helps to transfer the genes to the next generation, the soma of the organism is essentially disposable after reproduction. Why commit precious resources to a longer life, which doesn't help the genes move on? In certain cases, the best option is to get as many offspring as possible for the parent, and then die.

Another such example is the Pacific salmon; it reproduces once in its lifetime, and then dies. The salmon uses all of its reproductive energy, after which it appears to "simply fall apart." If there is no hope of a salmon surviving predators and other hazards to complete another round of reproduction, then it would not have been created by evolution to mature more slowly. Mice reproduce very prodigiously, attaining sexual maturity by age two. The mice devote more resources to reproduction than to counter the degradation of their bodies, subject to heavy predation.

But at the other hand, a longer life span could allow improved mechanisms to be built for repair. A 2-year-old mouse is ancient, while a 2-year-old elephant is just starting their lives. Less resources is devoted to growth in elephants, and they have much less offspring. An elephant's gestation period is eighteen to twenty-two months, and the result is only one living offspring. Mice grow in a litter up to fourteen young people, and can have five to ten litters a year.

While it is a useful concept, the disposable soma theory does have problems. This theory would suggest that intentional restriction of calories, which restricts overall resources, would result in less reproduction or a shorter life span. But calorie-restricted animals do not die younger— they live much longer, even to the point of near starvation. This influence is frequently seen in a number of different animal types. Depriving animals of food in turn allows them to devote more energy to combating aging.

Furthermore, most species females live longer than males. Disposable soma would expect the reverse, as females are expected to devote even more energy to reproduction and would thus have fewer time or resources to be allocated to sustain.

Verdict: This suits some of the evidence but it does have some significant issues. The theory of soma being disposable is either incomplete or incorrect.

FREE RADICAL THEORY

Biological processes create free radicals, which are molecules which can destroy the tissues around them. Cells neutralize them with antioxidants but this mechanism is incomplete, and damage accumulates over time, causing aging results. Large-scale clinical trials studies suggest that supplementing vitamins such as vitamin C and vitamin E with antioxidants may paradoxically raise mortality rates or contribute to worse health. Some factors known to better health or increase lifespan, such as calorie restriction and exercise, increase the development of free radicals, which function as signals to cells to upgrade their cellular defenses and mitochondria which generate energy. Antioxidants can abolish the effects of exercise which promote safety.

Verdict: Alas, certain details contradict the ideology of free radicalism. It, too, is either incorrect or incomplete.

MITOCHONDRIAL THEORY

Mitochondria are the energy-generating parts of the cells (organelles), and as stated earlier, they are also called the cells ' powerhouses. It's a tough work, and the mitochondria suffer a lot of molecular damage, so they need to be recycled and regularly replaced to maintain peak performance. Cells are autophagised; mitochondria have a common mechanism of replacing damaged organelles, called mitophagy. The mitochondria contain their own DNA which over time accumulates damage. The effect is weaker mitochondria, which in turn causes further damage in a process of viciousness. Cells will die without adequate energy, a manifestation of ageing.

Muscle atrophy is associated with elevated Mitochondrial damage rates. Yet little difference has been found in comparing energy output in the mitochondria among young and old people. For mice, very high mutation rates for mitochondrial DNA didn't contribute to accelerated aging.

Verdict: This is an interesting idea but it's really early and ongoing work. There can be reasons both for and against it.

HORMESIS

Mithridates VI was heir to Pontus, a area of Asia Minor, or modern-day Turkey, in 120 BC. His mother poisoned his father during a banquet, so that she might seize the throne. Mithridates walked north, living in the forest for seven years. He became chronically worried about being poisoned and took small doses of poison to make himself immune. He came back as a man to overthrow his mum and claim the throne. He was a mighty King. He resisted the Roman Empire during his rule but was incapable of pushing off the Romans. Through poison drinking Mithridates intended to commit suicide before his capture. "The Poison King" didn't die after taking massive doses, and the precise cause of his death is still uncertain. That which doesn't destroy you may actually make you stronger.

Hormesis is a process where low levels of stressors that are usually toxic actually strengthen an organism and make it more resistant to elevated levels of the same toxins or stressors. Fans of the film The Princess Bride can recall that for years the hero, Westley, had taken small doses of iocane powder which made him resistant to its toxic effects. So Westley was the only one to survive as Westley put the poison in both Vizzini's drink and his own. This is for hormesis.

Hormesis is not an aging hypothesis but has important consequences for other theories. The basic toxicological theory is "The dosage makes the poison." Low doses of "toxin" will make you safer.

Exercise and curbing calories are forms of hormesis. For example, exercise places stress on muscles which causes the body to respond by increasing muscle strength. Weight-bearing exercise puts stress on the bones, which causes the body to respond by increasing bone force. As astronauts do, being bedridden or moving into zero gravity causes the muscles and bones to quickly weaken.

Restriction of calories may be considered a stressor because it induces a increase in cortisol, widely known as the stress hormone.

This rise in cortisol increases heat shock protein production (a family of proteins that help stabilize new proteins or repair damaged ones) and tolerance to subsequent stressors. But calorie limitation also meets hormesis criteria. Since both exercise and calorie restriction are types of stress, they require free radical development.

Hormesis is no unusual phenomenon. For example, alcohol works through hormesis. Moderate alcohol intake is generally associated with improved health compared with total abstention. But heavy drinkers have poor health and the liver disease also develops. Exercise is well known to have positive health benefits but by triggering stress fractures, intense exercise can make health worse. Even small levels of radiation can enhance your health, whereas massive doses can kill you.

Many of the beneficial effects of certain foods may have been attributed to hormesis. Polyphenols are compounds in fruit and vegetables, coffee, chocolate and red wine, and they enhance health, likely in part by acting as low-dose toxins, thus upregulating the normal endogenous antioxidant enzymes throughout your body.

Why is hormone ageing important? Most aging theories presuppose all harm is negative and accumulates over time. But the hormesis hypothesis indicates that the body has potent potential for damage-repair which can be beneficial when triggered. Take training as an example. Weight lifting causes our muscles to get microscopic blood. That sounds pretty awful but they are made stronger by the act of rebuilding those muscles. Gravity fills our bones with pain. Weight-bearing activity like running allows our bones to get microfractures. Our bones are becoming stronger in the process of repair. In the zero gravity of outer space the same condition occurs. Bones are osteoporotic and weak without the force of gravity.

Not all damage is bad— in reality it is nice to have small doses of damage. What we're explaining is a regeneration process. Hormesis allows the breakdown of tissue such as the muscle or bone which is then rebuilt to be better able to withstand the stresses imposed on it. Muscles and bones will grow stronger but without breakdown and repair this development won't happen.

Verdict: Hormesis has ample evidence of being a true biological response to small doses of harm.

GROWTH VERSUS LONGEVITY

Hormesis, like the disposable soma hypothesis, implies that development and survival are essentially trade-offs. The larger an organism grows, the quicker it ages. Antagonistic pleiotropy may play a role in that certain genes that are beneficial in life early can be harmful in life later on. Comparing life spans within the same species, such as mice and dogs, means that smaller animals (those with less growth) live longer. Women, smaller on average than men, live longer, too. The shorter men live longer among men. Think of a 100 year old male. Imagine a 6-foot-6-inch muscular guy? Or do you just imagine a little man?

Nevertheless, larger animals live longer as compared across species. For example, the elephants live longer than mice. But the slower growth of larger animals may explain the difference. The relative absence of large animal predators has indicated that evolution has favored slower growth and a slower aging. Small animals often live longer, with less predators than other species of the same age, such as bats.

Aging is not engineered purposefully because the same physiological processes that drive development also cause aging. Aging is actually the continuation of the same growth plan and it is guided by the same nutrients and growth factors. When you rev the engine of a vehicle, high speeds can be achieved very easily but the engine must continue to run in burnout. It is the same program that is important, but different time scales— short-term success versus longevity. All ageing hypotheses point to this important trade-off. This is powerful knowledge, because at some times in our lives certain services can be beneficial. We need to develop, for example, during the youth. However, this high growth plan can cause premature ageing during the middle and older ages, and slow growth will be beneficial. Since the foods we consume play a significant role in this programming, we should make conscious changes to our diet in order to protect both our longevity and our "health period."

CHAPTER 2: AUTOPHAGY VERSUS CALORIES

In the expectation of living longer, the Calorie Restriction Society, which boasts more than 7,000 members, routinely believes in limiting calories. Sounds like a fantasy? Calorie restriction, with animal studies dating back several decades, may be the best represented among life-extension activities. Maybe the most effective antiaging technique currently known is calorie restriction (CR) with appropriate nutrition.

Studies of animals as early as 1917 show that restriction of calories can prolong life. Limiting the intake of food in young female rats delays menopause, leaving them even longer than average fertile. Researcher Clive McCay reported by 1935 that decreased growth of white rats caused by calorie restriction contributed to improved longevity. The animals should not be undernourished, however. Inadequate consumption of essential vitamins and minerals is responsible for many forms of diseases, and malnourished mice perform poorly and die early in general. Restricting energy (calories) while supplying all the necessary nutrients had the potential to prolong their life span, something unheard of previously.

Scientists usually used a calorie restriction of 40 per cent, but even a calorie restriction of 10 per cent in rats provides almost the same benefits. A 10 percent limit on calories improved life in these rats by about 15 percent, while animals that were limited by 40 percent lived about 20 years longer. Scientists first demonstrated in 1942 that calorie restriction in animals could prevent the cancer from growing. There are no regulated human trials available because ethically, they are almost impossible to conduct. We use the word calorie restriction for the remainder of the text, with the tacit assumption that malnutrition should be avoided.

Calorie restriction increases the life cycle of any organism studied so far, including yeast, worms, flies, rodents and monkeys. It also slows down or even eliminates age-related illnesses, including dementia, diabetes, cardiovascular and heart disease, neurodegenerative disorders, and multiple cancers. Scientists in 1946 insightfully observed that it would be difficult or even impossible to enforce a calorie-restricted diet in a abundant food climate, as the subsequent decades would show. Instead, they questioned whether with a periodic fasting schedule, a more practical type of calorie restriction could be enforced. Rat studies have shown that this technique has been effective in extending life and in preventing cancer.

Extending the concept to humans, Ross noted in 1959 the coronary heart disease is rare in populations with dietary deficiency. To put it another way, people consuming less calories tend to have less heart disease. Researchers have observed a lesser effect of protein restriction on longevity during this time span. In rat diets high casein (a type of dietary protein) shortens the lifespan.

Dr. Roy Walford was the leading promoter of calorie restriction for longevity at UCLA during the 1970's. Afterwards, he will become the Biosphere 2 physicist. This experimental project in the early 1990s was a self-contained greenhouse in which eight "Terranauts" lived in a fully sealed area. They were developing their own food and recycling the waste. They did not produce as much food as was originally expected, however. Dr. Walford convinced the other members of the team to complete their two-year task, adopting a calorie-restricted diet. Sadly, things have not gone exactly as he had expected. In addition to adopting a calorie-restricted diet, the

Terranauts were definitely not getting enough nutrition. Dr. Walford lost 25 pounds of his still spare 145-pound frame and came considerably aged out of Biosphere 2. He later acquired the disease of Lou Gehrig, and died at the age of 79.

In the 1980s, the calorie-restriction model was gradually embraced and considerable thought was given to how to adapt these animal experiments to humans. More and more academic publications are moving the knowledge limits on how calorie limitation can be a key component of longevity.

In the Japanese prefecture of Okinawa, one of the most convincing examples of calorie restriction in extending human life span is. The Okinawan people typically observe a custom called Hari Hachi Bu, which is a type of eating conscientiousness. The Okinawans are purposely told to avoid eating when they are 80 per cent loaded, essentially self-imposing a 20 per cent limit on calories. Among their population there are a whopping four to five times more centenarians than in most developed countries, and this phenomenon has been correlated with their low-calorie diets, which comprise around 20 per cent fewer calories than other Japanese citizens. This remarkable figure does not, however, apply to Okinawans who are younger than 65 years of age, which may be correlated with an increasingly Western-influenced diet that started to flow into their lifestyle in the 1960s.

Restriction of calories is the only non-pharmacological approach to reliably prolong the life span and defend against many age-related diseases. Animals, including humans, develop and grow when food is available but they also age rapidly. Both species have receptors of nutrients which are closely related to growth pathways. Once animals sense low nutritional supply, growth is turned all the way down, potentially triggering longevity pathways in the critical balance between development and longevity. Such control, of course, has its limits. Starvation and loss of the nutrients cause mortality and weakness. Yet calorie restriction is highly effective with optimum nutrient intake.

This paradigm shift is interesting on its surface. We just think of food as nourishment, but there should be more to it. Yet that is not so. Instead, depriving animals of food strategically does not reduce their life span; it increases them.

THE MECHANISMS OF CALORIE RESTRICTION

Originally, life extension definitions of calorie restriction sound extreme but studies have verified the relationship in several organisms several times over.

Essentially, slower development and reduced growth have contributed to longer life spans. Why? For what? There are several mechanisms working.

Low body fat may be the most obvious consequence of limiting chronic calories in animals but low visceral fat is of particular significance. High visceral fat accumulated in the abdomen and around major organs presents a significant health risk to humans and is strongly correlated with decreased sensitivity to insulin, obesity, type 2 diabetes, and atherosclerosis.

Genetically modified mice live longer on very low body fat. FIRKO (Knock Out Fat Insulin Receptor) mice have blocked insulin receptors. Since insulin usually tells the body to accumulate weight, these genetically modified mice can not become obese, and live longer than unchanged mice as well. All FIRKO and calorie-restricted mice have substantially decreased body fat, indicating that less body fat may be the common denominator extending life span.

But that's not the whole story as the health risks are often associated with being underweight or getting lower than average amounts of fat. There's one major mitigating factor here, though.

Individuals who are underweight may have secret diseases, such as cancer, which cause underweight, and it is unclear if intentionally reducing body fat below average is safe or harmful.

The metabolic rate declines with chronic calorie restriction. When you consume fewer calories your body will respond by burning fewer calories. This may not seem advantageous at first, but a lower metabolic rate correlates with less oxidative DNA damage, and thus may affect aging. Different animals have metabolic rates which vary widely. Generally speaking, the higher the metabolic rate, and the shorter the lives of animals, likely due to more free radical or oxidative harm. When the engine of your car is continuously revving, it can go quicker but burn out earlier. Higher levels of free triiodothyronine (T3), an essential metabolic-rate hormone, are associated with longer life in humans. Because the calorie restriction will lower the overall metabolic rate, energy consumption may be higher per gram of body weight. Some studies have shown that stable centenarians have both higher muscle mass and a higher metabolic rate which are associated with both.

NUTRIENT SENSORS

The longevity research still reverts to the competing desires of growth versus longevity. In general, higher growth results in lower longevity, and vice versa. Maximizing longevity therefore also depends on that growth, and one way we can influence that is through our nutrient sensors.

Primitive single-celled organisms live in a nutrient stream and, by halting development, can react quickly to a decrease in nutrient availability. For example, yeast and bacteria go into a dormant (spore) state that can live for thousands of years before reanimation when there is water and nutrients. When we became complex multicellular organisms, we always had to know if there were any nutrients there. We don't want to increase growth and metabolism during a time of drought, as that will rush our demise. Having a lot of kids during a famine could kill both mom and baby, which is why women without enough body fat stop ovulating. On the other hand, when food is abundant, our bodies need to stimulate growth pathways in order to evolve as soon as possible. Make hay as the saying goes when the sun shines. All animals ' survival depends on both providing nutrient sensors and closely connecting them to the growth pathways.

There are three recognized nutrient sensing pathways: insulin, mTOR (mechanical target of rapamycin), and AMPK (a protein kinase activated by AMP). Extending lifespan depends on decreasing growth and metabolism, which is best achieved by changing our diets by reducing the nutrient sensing pathways. The reduction of insulin (by reducing calories, but more importantly reducing refined grains and sugar), the reduction of mTOR (by reducing animal protein and using more plant proteins), and the activation of AMPK (by reducing calories) were all related to longevity.

INSULIN

The insulin hormone is the most well known transmitter of nutrients. Nutrition includes the three macronutrient mixtures: carbohydrates, protein, and fat. Our bodies respond to these macronutrients when we feed, by increasing the production of certain hormones. Insulin rises in response to carbohydrates and protein consumption, but dietary fat does not induce insulin secretion. Insulin enables the body's cells to use some ingested glucose for energy, acting on the GLUT4 protein. As such, insulin fulfills the function of a nutrient sensor by signalling to the rest of the body that certain nutrients are available.

But that's just one of the functions insulin plays. When insulin activates its cell surface receptor it also triggers the PI3 K pathway, resulting in protein synthesis and cell growth and division. This PI3 K activation occurs simultaneously and automatically because the nutrient sensors are inextricably connected to growth pathways. Insulin plays a role in both metabolism and development, which is generally highly beneficial to species survival because animals need to grow when food is available and stop growing when it is not available.

Animal studies show that higher availability of nutrients reduces life span. Add glucose to worm C diet. The elegants shorten their lives. The high glucose activates insulin and promotes development at the cost of a shortened life span. High levels of insulin and insulin resistance, normal in aging, have been consistently linked in humans to an increased risk of many age-related diseases, including cancer and heart disease.

The blood glucose and insulin levels decrease precipitously during calorie restriction and fasting. Lower insulin signaling reduces signaling for growth but increases life span in many animal species. Dismantling carbohydrates in the diet is another natural means of lowering insulin. Cynthia Kenyon, the scientist who discovered insulin and glucose functions in lifespan, considered the findings so convincing she was going on a low-carbohydrate diet. An essential factor in calorie restriction may be increasing insulin sensitivity and reducing insulin levels.

INSULIN-LIKE GROWTH FACTOR 1

Insulin-like growth factor 1, or IGF-1 is a hormone closely linked to insulin that plays a role in aging. Growth hormone (GH), which is secreted by the pituitary gland, was often assumed to be responsible for increasing children's development. The Israeli endocrinologist Zvi Laron founded the first pediatric endocrine clinic in that country in the 1950s. Several siblings with stunted growth were amongst his first patients. He thought they lacked GH but they were sky high when he tested their hormone levels. What happened? It would take several decades of study before we knew the answer.

Growth hormone acts to generate IGF-1 on its cell receptor, which is the actual mediator of the growth effect. The children Laron met, who suffered from what is now known as Laron dwarfism, had plenty of GH, but they did not develop IGF-1 because of a genetic defect in the receptor. The lack of IGF-1 accounted for the short stature of the babies. Solved mystery. Nonetheless, a discovery at the Laron dwarfs would later set the world of immortality on fire in 2013.

A band of about 300 members known as the Laron dwarfs lives in a remote corner of Ecuador. A community of Spanish Jews fled the Inquisition in the fifteenth century and hereditary inbreeding led to this group of people who lacked the hormone IGF-1 altogether. They grow to an average height of 4 feet but are usually established elsewhere. The local physician Dr. Guevara-Aguirre identified and followed this culture for many decades. He and his colleague from the University of Southern California, Dr. Valter Longo, made the surprising discovery that these Laron dwarfs appeared absolutely resistant to cancer! By contrast, unaffected members of these Laron dwarfs (those who don't have the syndrome) had a cancer rate of 20 percent.

Dr. Longo's interest in the less-growth longevity effect began in 2001 when he found that a long-lived yeast had the same form of growth pathway inhibition. Genetically deficient mice in growth hormone live 40 per cent longer— the 110-year human equivalent. Genetically modified animals have short lives despite the elevated growth hormone levels. Insulin and IGF-1 share many of the same features, and the receptor is similar in some animals. This result supports the idea that growth and longevity are essentially trade-offs.

mTOR

Another essential cellular nutrient sensor which is responsive to dietary proteins and amino acids is (mTOR) mammalian (or mechanistic) target of rapamycin. When you eat protein, it breaks down into its amino acid portion for bowel absorption, and increases mTOR. Eating enough protein to get the requisite amino acids is important for optimal safety, but avoiding excessive mTOR is also important for increasing the life span. Restriction of the dietary protein and fasting can reduce mTOR.

Like insulin, mTOR is a transmitter of nutrients and its activation is inextricably associated with growth pathways. When you sense protein supply your body will enter growth mode and start creating new proteins. This is an example of pleiotropic antagonism. During early life, mTOR encourages growth and development, but this process causes aging to damage us in later life. Any of the protein restriction benefits may be related to the impact mTOR has on autophagy.

Autophagy is a process of cellular recycling which breaks down old proteins and subcellular organelles. This cycle provides the required energy and amino acids to rebuild new proteins to replace the old proteins, which is a crucial factor in cell maintenance. Autophagy is the crucial first step in holding a cell in pristine condition, and aging is marked by a decrease in the rate of autophagy as damaged molecules accumulate in the cell and hinder its functioning. In rats, the difference between young and old animals is as much as six times that. Declining levels of autophagy mean damaged cell components such as lipid membranes and mitochondria are sticking around longer.

MTOR is the most active stimulus to turn off autophagy. Just a bit of the dietary protein increases mTOR, turning off autophagy and the process of cellular regeneration. Fasting significantly increases the rate of autophagy and is important in yeast for the life span–extending effects of calorie limitation. Drugs that block mTOR, such as rapamycin, can prolong the life span of yeast, largely due to its autophagy influence.

AMPK

The third nutrient sensor is called the protein kinase (AMPK) activated by the AMP. It acts as a sort of reverse fuel gage for stores of cellular energy. If you have plenty of energy in your car in the form of petrol, the scale reads big. If you have a lot of energy in your cells in the form of ATP (adenosine triphosphate) then AMPK is weak. Low levels of cellular energy push up levels of AMPK. AMPK thus serves as a kind of cellular fuel gauge except in reverse. Like mTOR and insulin, AMPK is linked to growth pathways by the nutrient sensor. AMPK down-regulates biological molecules synthesis including those required for growth (anabolism). Unlike insulin or mTOR, AMPK does not respond to any particular dietary macronutrient but assesses overall cellular energy availability.

Substances which activate AMPK (imitating low cellular energy stores) are known for health promotion. Examples include diabetes drug metformin, raisin and red wine resveratrol, green tea and dark chocolate epigallocatechin gallate (EGCG), pepper capsaicin, spice turmeric curcumin, garlic, and traditional Chinese medicinal herb berberine. Calorie restriction also activates AMPK, and the effects of AMPK on aging may be important to this fact.

AMPK improves glucose absorption into muscle cells, and increases mitochondrial production, resulting in increased fat burning efficiency. AMPK also increases autophagy, the important process of cellular self-cleaning which rides junk cells and recycles them, which we will discuss in more detail later.

Intermittent fasting, which implies going without food for some time, can have benefits for antiaging beyond pure limits on calories. There are several different rhymes for fasting. One common method includes a seventeen-hour fast (including sleeping time) and an eight-hour "feeding period." Some people practice alternate-day fasting, eating little or no food on one day, and eating is unrestricted on the following day.

Animals fed every other day, while eating about the same amount of food as regularly fed animals, behave physiologically like calorie-restricted animals. The animals who are fed every other day eat more on feeding days to counteract their days of fasting. This result casts some doubt as to whether less calories are necessary for the extension of the life span. Although total calories are identical between reducing calories and fasting every other day, the hormonal effects of fasting are quite different. All of the nutrient sensor pathways are engaged during fasting — insulin and mTOR decrease as AMPK increases. Certain hormones, called the counter-regulatory hormones, are growing. Such hormones include the hormones adrenaline, noradrenaline, and development. The increase in counter-regulatory hormones has the effect of rising energy and preserving basal metabolism. These hormonal shifts do not happen with a simple reduction in chronic calories. The calories may be the same but it's not the physiological effect. Reducing dietary fat, for example, decreases calories but not insulin or mTOR as the consumption of carbohydrates and proteins may remain the same.

Calorie-restricted (CR) animals are still hungry, leading to increased signals of hunger hormones. Since hunger is such a basic instinct, long-term denial of hunger is nearly impossible; hunger is dooming many weight-loss programs to failure. On the other hand, fasts also paradoxically decrease the cravings and desire for food. Many patients remember that hunger diminished by using intermittent weight loss fasting. They often comment that they felt their stomach shrank when, in fact, the signaling of hunger diminished.

Rats and mice that are put on a feeding / fasting scheme every other day live longer than fully fed animals. This result occurs without inherently reducing body weight, depending on the animal species used.

THE DOWNSIDES OF CALORIE RESTRICTION

Calorie restriction is only useful if the diet is sufficient. Calorie restriction may be taken too far. When a person falls below a certain body fat level, questions are posed about decreased immune function, low testosterone, feeling hungry and feeling cold. To the majority of Americans battling an obesity epidemic, these problems aren't big concerns. Perhaps the biggest thing with prolonged calorie restriction is that it's hard to manage. You need to scrupulously count every calorie. You have to prepare all of your meals. You need to measure the macronutrient ratios carefully to ensure you're getting enough of each. You must stop the fast food. Such things aren't easy to do and in many situations, not all of them can be done all the time. Calorie restriction operates only while the animals are locked in cages. It isn't working for the majority of people who have free will.

This is why scientists are so keen to discover the mechanisms of antiaging behind calorie restriction. By knowing those processes, we might replicate much of the advantages in twenty-first-century America in a realistic way that is consistent with daily life. There is clear evidence that less calories do not lie at the root of the advantages of the calorie restriction. Because the human body doesn't have calorie receptors or calorie counters, the benefits must be guided by hormonal shifts induced by dietary shift. Knowing these changes will lead us to naturally occurring "biohacks" (including modifying dietary protein and drinking coffee, tea and red wine, which we address further in the following chapters) that provide the same benefits.

CHAPTER 3: AUTOPHAGY FOR DETOX

Forget about tea cleanses and detox diets for the last time. They're words of plush nonsense. While there's certainly nothing wrong with drinking your weight in liquid salad, it's not going to flush out contaminants any faster than eating real food, you know.

The good news: The body cleanses itself in a little-known way, and it's a cycle you can manage.

You just have to practice a little self-cannibalism. What? What? Indeed, really, you can train your body to feed yourself — and believe it or not, you want it.

It is a normal mechanism called autophagy (literally "self-eating"), and it is the cleaning house method of the body: the cells build membranes that chase scraps of dead, diseased, or worn-out cells; suck them up; strip them for parts; and use the resulting molecules for energy or to produce new cell components.

"Think of it as the natural recycling system of our body," says Colin Champ, M.D., a board-certified oncologist for radiation, assistant professor at the University of Pittsburgh Medical Center and author of Misguided Medicine. "Autophagy allows us more effective machines to get rid of defective bits, stop cancerous growths and stop metabolic disease such as obesity and diabetes." There is also evidence that the cycle plays a role in regulating inflammation and immunity. And when scientists develop rats incapable of autophagy, they are fatter, sleepier, and have higher cholesterol and brain damage.

In short, autophagy is key to slowing down the aging cycle. And you can know better way to do it.

"So how do I eat myself?" is probably a question you haven't asked before, but we're about to tell you the answer. First of all, autophagy is a reaction to stress, so you're going to actually want to put your body through stress to drum up a little bit of extra auto-cannibalism. (We know this article is getting weirder, but trust us.) The autophagy detox process is caused by stressors on the body.

BENEFITS OF AUTOPHAGY

Autophagy is an extremely clever mechanism in which the body relies for cellular protection. Since it recycles old or damaged material, autophagy helps the body work during deprivation of nutrients (starvation, fasting, ketosis, etc). Essentially, during a time when no new protein is coming into the body, the body will use old proteins for food.

Autophagy also prevents toxic accumulation in the body of damaged cell components, especially mitochondria, and this induces cell death.

Autophagy has many other advantages: Promising Against Cancer

A 2012 study found autophagy to be an adaptable mechanism that can choose which materials to recycle depending on the type of stress the body is under. The study goes on to say that this adaptability makes autophagy an essential part of cancer-fighting and autophagy intervention may cause malignant illness. However, another study published in Clinical Cancer Research found that certain cancers are dependent on survival autophagy and that suppressing autophagy is a better treatment for those cancers. This information shows this is a complicated topic which needs further study.

Heart health

According to a study published in Circulation Cardiac disease induced by age is typically characterized by "hypertrophy, fibrosis, and accumulation of malfolded proteins and defective mitochondria." Autophagy is an important part of eliminating these defective materials but autophagy also decreases with age. Therefore, it makes sense that may autophagy may help improve heart problems related to ageing. The analysis shows how accurate this is. Deleting toxic materials in mouse experiments improves the cellular environment and therefore the wellbeing of the heart.

ALZHEIMER'S Autophagy is a vital mechanism for homeostasis of proteins and the protection of cells. Researchers and researchers are beginning to conclude that the autophagy deficiency in the body is likely to lead to neurodegenerative disorders like Parkinson's and Alzheimer's. Improving autophagy in the body may theoretically minimize or reverse the risk of developing Alzheimer's disease.

INCREASE LONGEVITY Autophagy is a mechanism of survival that allows people to live, and even succeed under stressful conditions. Autophagy can help to improve lifespan, because of this. But researchers are not fully clear about how longevity is influenced by autophagy, and conclude that further work is required to find out.

HOW TO INDUCE AUTOPHAGY Autophagy is triggered when the body is under adequate stress to create a biomechanical reaction. There are three main ways to do this: FASTING One way to cause autophagy is by limiting food for a certain amount of time. During this podcast segment, Day 3 and 4 of a water quick is when autophagy starts to kick during, according to Dr Daniel Pompa. When I was fasting a 7-day water (nothing but pure water), I found that 3-4 days I felt the worst, but soon after that I bounced back with a lot of strength.

There are some ways you can get some of the same benefits if you're not ready for a 3-7 day fast: INTERMITTENT FASTING–Intermittent fasting is when you eat less frequently (but no less food). When we are sleeping the night is already a time of fasting. Intermittent fasting extends out a little bit more time out. You could have dinner at 8 pm, for example, and not eat again until breakfast the next day at noon. Many experts say the eating the better the shorter the time. They recommend an eating window target of 4-8 hours.

TIME-RESTRICTED EATING (TRE) –It is very similar to intermittent fasting but also has an aspect of circadian rhythm. TRE supports feeding when the body is more capable of processing food (earlier in the day) and avoiding feeding by darkness as the body and metabolism wind down. With TRE a meal plan may be to eat dinner at 5 pm and not eat again until 8 am the next morning.

WORKING UP TO A FAST

You can work your way up slowly if you're nervous about jumping into a fast. The first step will be to eat 3 full meals a day, and avoid snacks. First, in a 4-8 hour eating period, you could try to make your fasting time longer (12 hours to get started) and theoretically reduce to two meals.

There are many ways to fast including juice fasting and broth fasting, but for the best results Dr. Pompa suggests a simple drink.

KETOSIS

While fasting has many advantages beyond triggering autophagy, it isn't always possible. Yet ketosis will carry many of the same advantages.

Ketosis is a condition in which the body uses fat rather than glucose as a fuel (like during fasting). Yet it can achieve ketosis without consuming all the food. Alternatively, like a ketogenic diet, you eat a high fat, moderate protein, low carb diet.

This form of diet eliminates calories, so that the body is forced to use fat for fuel again. Since fat burns cleaner than carbs and autophagy begin to work on recycling old stuff, ketosis entry can have a significant effect on cell health.

Dr. Pompa recommends you find something that fits for you. In certain individuals, a daily keto diet will not be feasible. He notes that some women think it works best if they eat more carbs during their period's week and then go back to a low carb diet afterwards. Others consider a keto diet six days a week and a carb day once a week helping to alleviate symptoms while supplying them with the same benefits of a keto diet.

How to Check

I used a meter like Keto Mojo to know for certain whether or not I am in ketosis. It detects a slight decrease in blood, and checks levels of blood ketone. Nutritional ketosis is known to be at rates of 0.5-1.5 mmol / L, and 1.5-3 mmol / L is considered suitable for fat burning and potentially autophagy.

As my body has adapted, I was able to quickly shift in and out of ketosis, even after a long fast overnight.

Exercise There are many benefits to exercise and it's no wonder that it can help cause autophagy, too. Researchers from a 2012 study explicitly believe that autophagy is responsible for the exercise's metabolic benefits. In body organs, exercise causes autophagy including muscle, liver, pancreas, and adipose tissue.

Exactly what sort of workout, and how much is most effective, is unclear. High-intensity interval training (HIIT) was shown to enhance withochondrial function, however. A research published in Aging further found that resistance training improved.

But any exercise should yield some profit, so just move on!

Sauna I've previously spoken about the health benefits of sauna use, and one reason it's so important is that it can induce autophagy. Work reported in Science Daily confirms that by triggering autophagy, the sauna will improve cellular health. The explanation is that the heat from a sauna creates some stress on the body which stimulates this process of detoxification.

BOTTOM LINE: AUTOPHAGY FOR DETOX

The body is complex, but incredible and intelligent. Autophagy is a great way for the body to adapt to combat stressors and improve cellular health. What's even more exciting about improving safety using autophagy is that it's open to all. No need to buy costly equipment or supplements! Autophagy inducing is as simple as creating small stressors which ultimately help to improve health.

CHAPTER 4: THE ART OF FASTING

Mentioning fasting as an obesity and type 2 diabetes treatment often receives the same eye-rolling response. Hunger? So, is that the answer? You going to starve people to death? No. No. It's not at all. I won't starve people; I'm asking them to fast.

Fasting in one key way is entirely different to starvation: energy. Starvation is the daily abstention from feeding. It is neither intentional nor regulated. Starving people have no idea when and where they will get their next meal. It happens in times of war and drought, where there is insufficient food. Fasting, on the other hand, is for moral, health or other purposes voluntary abstention from food. Food is available readily but you prefer not to consume it. No matter what the justification for abstaining, a vital difference is that fasting is voluntary.

Hunger and fasting should never be confused and the words should never be used interchangeably. Fasts and hungers exist on opposite sides of the planet. It's the difference between running and driving, when you're being chased by a lion. External powers force hunger upon you. Fasting, on the other hand, can be performed from a few hours to months on end for any period of time. You can start a fast at any time of your choosing, and you can also end a quick at will. For whatever reason, or for no reason at all, you can start or stop a fast.

Fasting doesn't have a traditional duration — because it's just the absence of food, you're basically fasting whenever you're not food. For example, the following day, a span of twelve hours or so, you could fast between dinner and breakfast. Fasting can be seen as a part of daily life in that context. Take the word breakfast. The word refers to the daily meal that "breaks your fast." The word itself clearly recognizes that fasting is performed everyday, far from being any form of cruel and unusual punishment, even if only for a short time. It's not a unusual thing but a part of everyday life.

Often I've found fasting the "old age" of weight loss. Why? For what? This is also an ancient method, going back thousands of years. Fasting is as ancient as history, far older than any other dietary strategy. But how does "secret" fast?

Though fasting was practiced for centuries, it was largely forgotten as a dietary therapy. There are virtually no books on that. A few websites are dedicated to fasting. Newspapers or magazines make almost no mention of it. Just its very description attracts incredulity stars. It is a safe spot in plain sight. How did they do this?

Big food corporations have been slowly transforming how we think about fasting through the influence about ads. Rather than being a purifying, balanced tradition, it is now seen as something to be feared and at all costs avoided. Fasting was incredibly bad for company, after all — selling food is hard if people are not going to eat. Fasting has been slowly but ultimately prohibited. Nutritional authorities now say that even missing a single meal would have serious implications for the safety.

Those messages are in books everywhere–on Television, in the newspaper. Hearing them over and over again generates the impression that they are certainly completely accurate and scientifically verified. The exact opposite is real. There is absolutely no connection between steady eating and good health.

Often the authorities will seek to persuade you, because you will be overwhelmed by hunger, that you can't easy. It's too hard. This really isn't possible. The reality here is the exact opposite too.

WHAT HAPPENS WHEN WE EAT?

We consume more food energy as we feed, than we can use instantly. Any of the energy has to be later put away. The main hormone involved in both food energy storage and use is insulin which rises during meals. Insulin is activated by both carbohydrates and by proteins. Fat causes a much smaller effect of insulin but it is rarely consumed alone.

Insulin has two main roles. Second, it lets the body start using food resources immediately. Carbohydrates are ingested and rapidly converted into glucose, which increases blood sugar levels. Insulin enables glucose to enter directly into most of the body's cells which use it for energy. Proteins are broken down and transformed into amino acids and excess amino acids can be converted into glucose, too. Protein does not increase blood glucose but can increase insulin levels. The effect is complex, and many people are shocked to learn that some proteins can activate insulin almost as much as certain foods containing carbohydrates. The fats are consumed directly as fat and have limited insulin effects.

Second, insulin helps to retain excess energy. There are two ways Energy can be stored. Glucose molecules can be fused together into long chains called glycogen and processed in the liver afterwards. But there is a limit to the quantity of glycogen that can be put away. When the limit has been hit, the body starts to turn glucose into fat. This cycle is known as de novo lipogenesis (literally, "making new fat").

This newly produced fat can be contained in the liver or in body fat deposits. Although converting glucose into fat is a more complicated process than storing it as glycogen, the amount of fat that can be produced is not limited.

What Happens When We Fast?

When we fast, the cycle of using and storing food energy that takes place when we eat goes in reverse. The levels of insulin go down, allowing the body to start consuming stored fat. Glycogen (the glucose that is contained in the liver) is the most readily available source of sugar, and the liver retains enough sugar for about twenty-four hours. The body then starts breaking down stored body fat for energy.

So you see, the body actually only exists in two states— the state of fed (high-insulin) and the state of fasted (low-insulin). Either we store the energy for food or we use the energy for food. If there is a balance between feeding and fasting, otherwise there is no net weight gain.

However, if we spend most of the day storing food resources (because we are in the fed state), then we'll gain weight over time. What is then required is to restore equilibrium by the the amount of time we consume food energy (by entering the fasted state).

The transformation from the fed state to the fasted state takes place in several stages, as one of the leading experts in fasting physiology, George Cahill, has described classically: 1. Feeding: Blood sugar levels are increasing as we consume the incoming food, and insulin levels are rising in response to transferring glucose into cells that use it for energy. Excess glucose is processed in the liver as glycogen, or converted into fat.

2. The post-absorptive process (six to twenty-four hours after starting fasting): Blood sugar and insulin levels are beginning to drop at this stage. The liver begins breaking down glycogen to supply energy, releasing glucose. Glycogen stores last for twenty-four to thirty-six hours.

3. Gluconeogenesis (twenty-four hours to two days after start of fasting): Glycogen stocks are running out at this stage. The liver produces new amino acid glucose in a cycle known as

gluconeogenesis (literally, "making new glucose"). Glucose levels decline in nondiabetic individuals but remain within normal limits.

4. Ketosis (two to three days after the start of fasting): Low levels of insulin induce lipolysis, fat breakdown for energy. Triglycerides, the fat type used to store them, are broken into the backbone of glycerol and three chains of fatty acids. The glycerol is used for gluconeogenesis, and the previously used amino acids can be reserved for protein synthesis. Most tissues in the body use the fatty acids directly for energy, but not the brain. The body uses fatty acids to create ketone bodies which can cross the blood-brain barrier and are used for energy by the brain. Following four days of fasting, ketones supply about 75 percent of the energy the brain uses. The two main types of ketones released are beta-hydroxybutyrate and acetoacetate, which during fasting may increase by more than seventy times.

5. The protein conservation process (five days after fasting starts): High growth hormone levels preserve muscle mass and lean tissues. Fatty acids and ketones provide nearly all of the energy for essential metabolism. Glyconeogenesis is used to control blood glucose using glycerol. Increased levels of norepinephrine (adrenaline) avoid any decrease in metabolic rate. A normal amount of protein turnover exists but it is not used for energy.

In essence the cycle of transitioning from burning glucose to burning fat is what we are explaining here. Fat is essentially the energy contained in the body's food. In periods of low supply of food, processed food is released to fill the gap, naturally. In an attempt to feed itself, the body does not "destroy food" until all the fat reserves are used up.

One important point to emphasize is that these processes are totally natural and fully regular. Low-availability cycles have always been a natural part of human evolution, and our bodies have evolved mechanisms to adapt to this Paleolithic fact of life. Otherwise we as a group wouldn't have existed. There are no adverse health effects for triggering such protocols, except for malnutrition (you shouldn't run if you are undernourished, of course, and excessive fasting may also trigger malnutrition). The body doesn't "shut down;" it's simply shifting sources of fuel, from food to our own fat. It does so with the aid of several hormonal fasting adaptations.

BENEFITS FOR ATHLETES

Many of these hormonal shifts may be of particular benefit to athletes. First of all, their net physiological effect is to retain lean mass (muscle and bone) over the duration of fasting, which has major implications for athletes. Second, although few studies, the higher level of growth hormone can boost the recovery time from hard workouts. The increased adrenaline also helps the workout to be more intense. Athletes can practice harder to get back up faster. Most elite athletes are becoming more interested in the benefits of "fasted state training." It's not by mistake that many of the early supporters of fasted state training are bodybuilders. In particular, this is a sport that requires high-intensity training and extremely low body fat. Both are bodybuilders: Brad Pilon, author of Feed, Stop, Sleep, and Martin Berkhan, who popularized the LeanGains fasting process.

The Importance of Healthy Eating

Fasting is not, of course, a cure-all-healthy eating is still important.

The greatest problems in modern medicine are metabolic diseases: obesity, type 2 diabetes, high blood pressure, elevated blood cholesterol and fatty liver, known collectively as metabolic syndrome. The involvement of each of these diseases raises enormously the risk of heart disease, stroke, cancer and premature death. And the origins of metabolic syndrome are in the Western diet, with its excess of sugar, high fructose corn syrup, artificial flavours, artificial sweeteners and overdependence on processed grains.

Those metabolic disorders do not impact populations that have maintained their conventional eating habits. This book focuses on one specific aspect of conventional eating habits in today's culture that is largely forgotten: intermittent fasting. This, however, is only part of the solution. It's not enough to simply add fasting to your life for optimum safety. You will need to focus on balanced eating habits.

What "healthy eating" does not mean is that there is a tendency to describe a balanced eating pattern as just any macronutrient mix. Only three macronutrients exist: carbohydrates, proteins, and fats. Many expert-recommended "balanced" diets specify some percent of these three — for example, the older American Dietary Guidelines suggested that dietary fat be kept to less than 30 percent of total calories. Unfortunately, the widespread acceptance of diet and calorie labeling on packaged food has added to that perception.

While this may sound empirical, these guidelines are not based on any specific basis. The basic premise of the recommendations based on macronutrients is that all fats are equal, all carbohydrates are equal and all proteins are equal. This, however, is simply wrong. Extra virgin olive oil, though both are pure fat, is not the same as trans-fat-laden margarine. Our bodies react to each in a completely different way. Wild salmon protein isn't the same as highly processed gluten (which is a protein although present in grains). Sugar-derived carbohydrates are not the same as broccoli or kale carbohydrates. White bread is not similar to white beans. Differences in the way our bodies metabolize these various foods are easy and easily observable.

The same is true with respect to calories. Dietary recommendations defining calorie limits unwittingly presume that all calories are equal, but one hundred calories of a green salad as one hundred calories of chocolate chip cookies do not have the fattening impact.

Relying on recommendations focused on macronutrients or calorie caps makes eating much more difficult than it should be. We are not consuming a specific amount of fats, protein and carbohydrates. We eat groceries. Some foods are more abrasive than others. So the safest recommendation is to consume or not consume particular foods, not particular nutrients.

Considering that chronically high levels of insulin are the root cause of all metabolic syndrome diseases, it is especially important for those with metabolic syndrome to understand how foods induce insulin release. Fasting is of course the greatest tool in your arsenal when it comes to lowering insulin levels— since all foods activate insulin to some degree, consuming none at all is the safest way to lower insulin. We can not accelerate forever however, so there are some basic rules to obey to lower insulin rates.

EAT WHOLE, UNPROCESSED FOODS

Human beings evolved to eat a wide range of foods with no negative health effects. Traditionally, the Inuit people eat exceptionally high diets in animal products, indicating high amounts of fat and protein. Many, like the Okinawans, eat a conventional root vegetable-based diet, meaning it's high in carbohydrates. Yet, historically, both groups did not suffer from metabolic diseases. This only emerged when their diets became increasingly westernised.

What mankind has not evolved to consume is highly processed food. The normal balance of macronutrients, fiber, and micronutrients is completely broken during processing. Of example, wheat berry processing to eliminate all of the fat and protein ensures the product, white flour, is almost pure carbohydrates. Wheat berries are natural; this is not white flour. This is also grounded to an extremely fine consistency which greatly speeds up carbohydrate absorption into the bloodstream. And other grains produced experience the same problems. Our body has evolved to manage natural food and the effect is sickness when we feed it on artificial foods.

Imagine a beautiful red Ferrari sports car sitting at the driveway. Suppose instead that we "process" it by removing the doors and wheels from a truck and inserting bicycle tires and rusty blue doors. Is it the same wagon? Neither at all.

There's nothing inherently bad about foods that contain carbohydrates. The problem occurs when we begin to shift certain foods from their natural state and then eat them in large quantities. The same goes for refined fats too. Processing turns fairly harmless vegetable oils into fats containing trans-fats, contaminants which have now become well established as hazards.

Foods in their natural state would be identifiable as something that was alive or that has come out of the earth. Cheerios boxes aren't rising in the forest. This can be stopped if it comes prepackaged in a bag or box. This can be stopped because it has a warning mark. Organic products have no names, be they broccoli or beef.

The true secret to eating good is this: eat real food only.

REDUCE SUGARS AND REFINED GRAINS

For certain reasons it is best to avoid all processed foods, but not always 100 per cent possible. So it's necessary to know which foods are the biggest criminals, so we can stop them.

For anyone, but particularly those with metabolic syndrome, avoiding sugars and refined grains, such as meal and corn products, is most important. These are more fattening than other foods, even though they have the same amount of calories, which is why low-carbohydrate diets are good for losing weight.

EAT MORE NATURAL FATS

Diät fat has been considered number one public enemy for several decades. (We can speak further about the myths behind low-fat diets for weight loss and heart safety. Slowly, health officials have come to understand that it has been wrongly targeted. However, while the word "good fats" was once considered an oxymoron, it is now just a well-accepted fact of life. Foods rich in monounsaturated fats, such as olive oil, nuts and avocados, which were previously pre-saturated.

EAT LESS ARTIFICIAL FATS

But not all the fats are so harmless. Partially hydrogenated vegetable oils, used in products such as shortening, deep-fried meats, margarine, and baked goods such as cakes and cookies, contain trans-fats that are not treated well by our bodies. Trans-fats elevate cholesterol LDL ("bad") and lower cholesterol HDL ("good"), raising the risk of heart disease and stroke.

Highly refined vegetable oils such as corn, sunflower, and canola oils were once considered "heart safe." Maize oil, for example, for a natural fat, is easy to confuse. But in reality, corn is not oily by definition. To fill the bottle of corn oil you can buy in the supermarket so easily it needs literally grinding tons of corn. And as it turns out, recent studies show very high levels of these oils in inflammatory omega-6 fats. Although some omega-6 fats are required, we are likely to consume ten to twenty times as many as we have in the past, and when our intake of omega-6 fats is out of balance with our intake of omega-3 fats (found in fatty cold-water fish, nuts and seeds), the result is systemic inflammation, which is a concern in heart disease, type 2 diabetes, inflammatory intestinal disease and other chronic diseases.

Eating healthy fats and avoiding unhealthy fats, such as partially hydrogenated oils and heavily refined vegetable oils, is essential to good health.

DIFFERENT KINDS OF FASTING

There are several different ways to accelerate and there is no "right" way to do that. An utter fast deprives both food and air. This can be achieved for religious reasons, as in the Muslim tradition during the holy month of Ramadan. No food or beverage is consumed during the period between sunrise and sunset during that time.

Medically this combines fasting dietary restriction with dehydration due to fluid restriction. It raises the physical complexity of an absolute quick and restricts the length to relatively short periods. For safety reasons absolute fasts are not commonly recommended. The resulting dehydration does not offer any extra health benefits to counter the increase in difficulty. At utter fasts, too, the chance of medical problems is much higher.

Earlier in the book we'll explore a number of specific fasting schedules. Intermittent fasting can be enforced effectively with either quick fasts (less than 24 hours) or longer fasts (more than 24 hours). You can also safely use prolonged fasting (more than three days) for weight loss and other health benefits.

THE ADVANTAGES OF FASTING

Fasting's most obvious benefit is weight loss. However, there are a myriad of benefits beyond this, many of which were widely known before the modern era. It was once common for people to fast for a certain period of time for health benefits. These fasting periods were often called "cleanses," "detoxifications," or "purifications," and people believed that they would clear their bodies of toxins and rejuvenate them. They were more correct than they knew. Fasting:

Improves mental clarity and concentration

Induces weight and body fat loss

Lowers blood sugar levels

Improves insulin sensitivity

Increases energy

Improves fat-burning

Lowers blood cholesterol

Prevents Alzheimer's disease

Extends life

Reverses aging process

Decreases inflammation

We'll talk more about these health benefits in later chapters. But why is fasting better than other diets? We'll look at the advantages to fasting in this chapter.

Diets Fail

One main problem of the diets that have the health benefits listed above is that these are often very difficult to follow, as I discovered when working with my patients with obesity and type 2 diabetes.

Obesity and type 2 diabetes are both problems of excessive insulin. Since refined carbohydrates are a prime contributor to high insulin levels, the natural place to start with my patients was a low-carbohydrate diet. Protein, especially animal proteins (dairy and meat), can also stimulate insulin production, and excessive intake of these foods can slow down progress. And processed foods also play a key role in disease. So, the best diet would emphasize whole, unprocessed foods. It would be low in refined carbohydrates and high in natural fats with a moderate amount of protein.

Multiple peer-reviewed studies have shown that that kind of diet has excellent results for type 2 diabetes and is very safe. So that's what I started with in working with my patients at the Intensive Dietary Management Program. I counseled them on reducing sugars and refined carbohydrates and replacing them with natural, unprocessed foods. I gave lectures. I followed up. I begged. I cajoled. I reviewed page after page of food diaries. *And it just did not work.*

The diet could be successful, but only if it was properly followed, and it was simply too complicated for many of my patients. They would return food diaries filled with noodles and bread and still claim they were following a low-carbohydrate diet. Pitas, naan, and other flatbreads somehow were not considered "bread." They simply did not understand what was being asked of them. These were not, after all, people obsessed with nutrition who spent every spare minute reading medical journals. They had full-time jobs and families to take care of, and trying to break their dietary habits of the last fifty years proved to be very challenging. Also, because this diet was almost the opposite of conventional dietary advice, it was often hard for people to accept that it was actually good for them.

But I couldn't just give up. Their health and, indeed, their very lives depended upon the proper treatment. Type 2 diabetes is a terrible disease. It is by far the leading cause of blindness, amputation, and kidney failure in North America. Diabetes is also a leading contributor to heart attacks, stroke, and other cardiovascular diseases. Type 2 diabetes is a dietary disease, and it requires a dietary solution. Most importantly, it is a *curable* disease.

What I needed was a new strategy. The overall goal was not necessarily to reduce carbohydrate intake. The goal was to reduce insulin levels, and cutting carbohydrates was only one method of achieving that goal. Yet all foods, to varying degrees, stimulate the release of insulin. So the most efficient method of lowering insulin would be to eat nothing at all. In other words: to fast.

I didn't need to reinvent the wheel. People are always drawn to the latest and greatest diet trend, the next superfood, like quinoa, acai berries, or kale chips. But what are the chances that, after thousands of years of human history, we will find the "next great thing" now? The thing that we can't live without, despite having lived without it for thousands of years?

Fasting is the oldest dietary intervention in the world. It is profoundly different from all other dietary strategies. It is not the latest and greatest but the tried and true. It is not something to do but something to *not* do. Because it differs from conventional dieting in many important ways, fasting carries many distinct advantages.

ADVANTAGE #1: IT'S SIMPLE

Because there is no consensus as to what constitutes a healthy diet, my patients were often confused. Should they go low-fat? Low-carb? Low-calorie? Low-sugar? Low glycemic index?

Fasting is much easier to understand, when following a completely different approach. It's so easy it can be explained in two phrases: Eat nothing. Drink soda, coffee, tea, or bone bread. That's it.

ADVANTAGE #2: IT'S FREE

I prefer patients to eat organic, local grass-fed beef and organic vegetables, and avoid white bread and other highly processed foods. However, the truth is that these kinds of healthy foods are often very expensive; they can cost ten times as much as processed foods.

Grains enjoy substantial government subsidies, making them far cheaper than other foods. This means that a pound of fresh cherries may cost $6.99, while an entire loaf of bread will cost $1.99. An entire box of pasta may cost only $0.99 on sale. Feeding a family on a budget is a lot easier when you buy pasta and white bread.

If a diet is unaffordable, it does not truly matter if it is effective. The price makes it ineffective for those who cannot afford to follow it. This should not doom them to a lifetime of type 2 diabetes and disability.

Fasting is free. In fact, not only is it free, it actually saves money because you do not need to buy any food at all! Food is not costly. There are no costly add-ons. There are no bars, drinks, or drugs to cover meals. Fasting price is zero.

ADVANTAGE #3: IT'S CONVENIENT

It is healthy to always eat a home-cooked, prepared-from-scratch meal. However, many people, myself included, simply do not have the time or inclination to cook. Between work, school, family, kids, after-school activities, and after-work activities, there just is not a lot of time left over. Cooking involves preparation time, shopping time, cooking time, and cleanup time. Everything takes time, and time seems to be one commodity that's in constant shortage.

The number of meals eaten away from home has been steadily increasing over the past few decades. While many try to support the "slow food" movement, it is clear that they are fighting a losing battle against fast food.

So asking people to devote themselves to home cooking, as well-intentioned as it may be, is not going to be a winning strategy. Fasting, on the other hand, is the exact opposite. There is no time spent buying groceries, preparing ingredients, cooking, and cleaning up. It is a way to simplify your life.

There is nothing easier than fasting, because fasting involves doing nothing. Most diets tell you what to do. Fasting tells you not to do anything. It doesn't get easier than that.

ADVANTAGE #4: YOU CAN ENJOY LIFE'S LITTLE PLEASURES

Some diets advise people to never, ever again eat ice cream or desserts. Good advice for weight loss, obviously. But I don't think it is actually very practical advice. Sure, you might be able to swear off desserts for six months or a year, but for life? And would you really want to? Think about it. Imagine the joy of savoring the cake and champagne at your best friend's wedding. Do we need to deny ourselves that little bit of pleasure forever? Enjoy a birthday salad instead of birthday cake? Thanksgiving kale chips! All-you-can-eat Brussels sprouts! Yes, life just got a little less sparkly. Forever is a long time.

Now, I am not saying that you should eat dessert every single day. However, fasting restores the ability to occasionally enjoy that dessert by balancing out the feast. It is, after all, the cycle of life. Feasts follow fasts. Fasts follow feasts. This is how we have always lived. Birthdays, weddings, holidays, and other special occasions have always, throughout human history, been celebrated with feasts. But those feasts should be followed by fasts.

If you have a wedding coming up, you are more than entitled to look forward to enjoying yourself and eating decadent, delicious wedding cake. And when you fast regularly, you do not need to feel guilty about enjoying one of life's little pleasures, because you can make up for it.

The most important aspect of fasting is fitting it into your life. There will be times where it is not appropriate to fast. Who wants to forever be the party pooper who won't eat this and won't drink that? You can indulge yourself, as long you balance that with some abstinence. Fasting is really about *balance*. It is the flip side, the B-side, of eating. Balance the time that you are eating and the time you are not eating to remain healthy. When those two fall out of balance, that's when we get into trouble.

ADVANTAGE #5: IT'S POWERFUL

Many type 2 diabetics are morbidly obese and highly insulin-resistant. Occasionally, even a strict ketogenic diet (one that's very low in carbohydrate, moderate in protein, and high in fat) is not strong enough to reverse their disease. The quickest and most efficient way to lower insulin and insulin resistance is fasting. It has unrivaled power to break through weight-loss plateaus and reduce the need for insulin.

From a therapeutic standpoint, a key advantage of fasting is that it has no upper limit—there's no maximum amount of time that you can fast. The world record for fasting was 382 days, during which the patient suffered no ill effects. So if fasting occasionally isn't working, all you need to do is increase the frequency or length of time you fast, until you reach your goal.

Compare this to medications. Virtually every drug has a maximum dose. If you take penicillin for an infection, for example, there is a maximum dose above which there is little extra benefit and the medication may become toxic. At that point, if you still have the infection, you need to change medications. The same applies to low-carbohydrate or low-fat diets. Once you hit zero carbs or fat, you can go no further with that diet. There is a maximum dose. Once you reach the maximum, you need to change diets to gain any extra effect.

Advantage #6: It's Flexible

Some diet plans advocate eating as soon as you wake up and then every two and a half hours during the day. Some people have had good results with such a diet. However, finding or packing something to eat six or seven or eight times a day is very intrusive. I could not imagine interrupting my life every two and a half hours to snack. It's too disruptive on an already hectic schedule. And it's simply not necessary.

Fasting can be done at any time. There is no set duration. You may fast for sixteen hours or sixteen days. You can mix and match time periods. You are never locked into a pattern. You may fast for one day this week, five days the next, and two days the week after. Life is unpredictable. Fasting fits wherever you need it to.

Fasting can be done anywhere. It does not matter if you live in the United States, the United Kingdom, or the United Arab Emirates. You may live in the polar desert of the Arctic or the sandy desert of Saudi Arabia. It matters not at all. Once again, because fasting is about *not* doing something, it simplifies our life. It adds simplicity where other diets add complexity.

When for whatever reason you're not feeling good, you literally stop fasting. It is completely reversible in minutes. If for personal or medical purposes you want to stop fasting for many weeks then you might want to do so. If you want to treat yourself during the Christmas holidays or a summer cruise, you can do that too. Only get back on the track once you're done.

Compare this with bariatric surgery (sometimes called "stapling the stomach"). This has helped a lot of people lose weight, in the short term at least. But there are plenty of complications in this surgery which are almost all irreversible. And you simply can not undo the process itself. It is eternal. If you're doing poorly, then that's just too bad. Fasting, on the other hand, is completely beyond your control; you can speed or avoid fasting whenever you wish.

Fasting can be flexible. The day of a fast can be moved around and doesn't have to be set in stone. If I've got a particularly important meeting on a Thursday, for example—and feel it would be best to eat a breakfast—I can either change the hours I fast or just move it to another day in the week.

Advantage #7: It Works with Any Diet

Here is the biggest advantage of all: fasting can be added to any diet. That is because fasting is not about something you do; it's about something you do *not* do. It is subtraction rather than addition. This makes fasting fundamentally different from almost every diet imaginable.

You don't eat meat? You can still fast.

You don't eat wheat? You can still fast.

You have a nut allergy? You can still fast.

You don't have time? You can still fast.

You don't have money? You can still fast.

You are traveling all the time? You can still fast.

You don't cook? You can still fast.

You are eighty years old? You can still fast.

You have problems chewing? You can still fast.

What could possibly be simpler?

FASTING FOR A CLEANER BODY AND MIND

The most obvious advantages of fasting are that it helps with losing weight and type 2 diabetes, but there are many other benefits, including autophagy (a method of cell cleansing), lipolysis (fat-burning), anti-aging effects, and neurological benefits. Fasting, in other words, will support your brain and help keep your body younger.

Boosting Brainpower

Mammals generally respond to severe caloric deprivation by reducing organ size, with two prominent exceptions: the brain and, in males, the testicles. Reproductive function is preserved to propagate the species. But cognitive function is just as important and also highly preserved, at the expense of every other organ.

This makes a lot of sense from an evolutionary standpoint. Suppose food is scarce and difficult to find. If cognitive function started to decline, the mental haze would make it that much harder to find food. Our brainpower, one of the main benefits we have in the natural world, would be squandered. So what actually happens during caloric deprivation is that the brain maintains or even boosts its abilities. The best-selling novel *Unbroken*, by Laura Hillenbrand, describes the experiences of American prisoners of war in Japan during World War II. During their extreme starvation, the prisoners experienced some astonishing mental clarity that they themselves understood was due to the effect of starvation. One man was able to learn Norwegian in just under a week. Another described "reading" entire books from memory.

Originally, I was interested in the fasting research that demonstrated a reduction in inflammation and increase in growth hormone. However, when I began fasting through the morning, I immediately noticed a significant increase in mental focus, energy, and productivity. As a brain science geek, I'm impressed by the mental benefits of fat-adaptation and intermittent fasting.

Humans, like all mammals, have an increase in mental activity when hungry and a decrease when satiated. We have all experienced a "food coma"— think about how you feel after a big Thanksgiving meal, complete with turkey and pumpkin pie. Are you mentally sharp as a tack? Or dull as a concrete block? Despite popular belief, it's not the tryptophan in the turkey causing that postprandial drowsiness—in fact, turkey has about the same amount of tryptophan as other poultry. It's just the sheer amount of food. As the amount of blood going to the digestive system is increased to handle all that turkey and pie, less blood is available to go to the brain. About the only mental challenge we can handle after that enormous meal is sitting on the couch watching football.

How about the opposite? Think about a time that you were really, really hungry. Were you tired and sluggish? I doubt it. You were probably hyperalert, your senses sharp as a needle. Animals that are cognitively sharp and physically agile during times of food scarcity have a clear advantage when it comes to survival. If missing a single meal reduced our energy and mental acuity, we would have even more trouble finding food, making it more likely that we would go hungry again, leading to a vicious cycle ending in death. That's not, of course, what happens. Our ancient ancestors grew more alert and active when hungry so that they could find their next meal —and the same thing still happens to us.

Even our language reflects the relationship between hunger and mental acuity. When we say we are hungry for something—hungry for power, hungry for attention—does it mean we are slothful and dull? No, it means that we are on our toes, alert and ready for action. Fasting and hunger energize us and activate us to advance towards our goal, despite popular misconceptions to the contrary.

In one study of mental acuity and fasting, none of the factors measured—including sustained attention, attentional focus, simple reaction time, and immediate memory—were found to be impaired. Another study of two days of almost total caloric deprivation found no detrimental effect on cognitive performance, activity, sleep, and mood.

That's what happens to our brains during fasting. But the neurological benefits of fasting aren't limited to the times when we're actually forgoing food. Animal studies show that fasting has remarkable promise as a therapeutic tool. Aging rats started on intermittent fasting regimens markedly improved their motor coordination, cognition, learning, and memory. Interestingly, there was even increased brain connectivity and new neuron growth from stem cells. A protein called brain-derived neurotrophic factor (BDNF), which supports the growth of neurons and is important for long-term memory, is believed to be responsible for some of these benefits. In animals, both fasting and exercise significantly increase the beneficial BDNF effects in several parts of the brain. Compared to normal mice, mice on an intermittent fasting regimen showed less age-related deterioration of neurons and fewer symptoms of Alzheimer's disease, Parkinson's disease, and Huntington's disease.

Human studies on caloric reduction find similar neurologic benefits—and since fasting certainly restricts calories, this is one area where fasting and caloric reduction provide similar benefits. With a 30 percent reduction in calories consumed, memory significantly improved and the synaptic and electrical activity in the brain increased.

In addition, insulin levels have an inverse correlation to memory—that is, the lower the insulin level, the more memory improves. On the flip side, a higher body mass index is linked to decline in mental abilities and decreased blood flow to those areas of the brain involved in attention, focus, reasoning, and more complex, abstract thought. So fasting provides neurological benefits two ways: it decreases insulin and leads to consistent, maintained weight loss.

SLOWING AGING

When you buy a new car, everything works great. But after a few years, it starts to get a little beat up and needs more maintenance. You need to replace the brake pads, then the battery, then more and more parts. Eventually, the car is breaking down all the time and costing thousands of dollars to maintain. Does it make sense to keep it around? Likely not. So you get rid of it and buy a snazzy new car.

Important work tends to suggest a drastic decrease in inflammation, changes in insulin signaling and a near-total "reset" in immune function with 3–5-day fasts. It appears that abnormal and even pre-cancerous cells are forced towards apoptosis, which ultimately selects healthy cell types. In general, this represents a mechanism that would (theoretically) reverse many of the signs and symptoms of aging and at the same time that the mechanisms that tend to be involved in autoimmune and cancer.

Through that sense the body's cells are like vehicles. Subcellular sections need to be removed and replaced as they mature, and ultimately a cell is too old to repair and needs to be killed to make room for a fresh new cell.

Cells that reach a certain age are programmed to commit suicide in a cycle called apoptosis, also known as programmed cell death.

Although this may at first sound like a macabre, the cycle is continuously renewing cell populations making it important for good health. So when you need to remove only a few cellular components, a cycle called autophagy kicks in.

The term autophagy, coined by Christian de Duve, the Nobel Prize winning scientist, derives from the Greek auto ("self") and phagein ("eat"). Autophagy is a type of cellular cleaning: it is a controlled, organized process of breaking down and recycling cellular components when there is no longer enough energy to sustain them. When all the diseased or broken-down cellular parts have been washed, the body will begin the renovation process. New tissues and cells are being created to replace the ones killed. The body renews itself in this way. But this only works when the old pieces are first discarded.

Our bodies are in a state of continuous regeneration. Although we often concentrate on new cell growth, we often forget that the first step in regeneration is to remove the old cellular machinery that is broken down. But both apoptosis and autophagy are required to maintain our bodies in good working order. Diseases such as cancer occur when these mechanisms are disrupted, and the accumulation of older cellular components may be responsible for many of the consequences of aging. If autophagocytic processes are not regularly triggered, these undesirable cellular components build up over time.

Higher glucose levels, insulin levels, and proteins all toggle off autophagy. And it doesn't need a number. Although as little as three grams of the leucine amino acid will avoid autophagy. Here's how it works: The rapamycin (mTOR) pathway mammalian target is an essential sensor of nutrient availability. When we eat carbohydrates or protein, insulin is secreted and the increased amounts of insulin, or even just the amino acids from the ingested protein breakdown, activate the mTOR pathway. The body senses that food is available, and determines that there is no need to remove the old subcellular machinery as there is plenty of energy to go around. The end product of this is autophagy suppression. In other words, excessive food consumption, such as all day snacking, suppresses autophagy.

Conversely, autophagy is encouraged when mTOR is dormant—when it is not activated by elevated amounts of insulin or amino acids from ingested food. As the body detects the temporary absence of nutrients, it must give priority to the cellular sections to preserve. The oldest and most worn-out cellular parts are discarded, and amino acids from the broken-down cell parts are distributed to the liver, which uses them during gluconeogenesis to produce glucose. They can also be found in new proteins. It is important to remember that mTOR's dormancy is only related to the availability of short-term nutrients and not the presence of stored energy, such as liver glycogen or body fat. Whether the body has sufficient energy for mTOR and thus autophagy is irrelevant.

For people with chronic inflammatory and/or neurological conditions, fasting can help accelerate autophagy and the body's clearing-out of old, damaged tissue. The body engages in "housecleaning" all the time, but when it gets a break from the constant digestion of large amounts of food, it may be able to focus more energy on repair and restoration.

This is why the strongest stimulus to autophagy currently known is fasting, and why fasting alone, unique among diets, stimulates autophagy—simple caloric restriction or dieting isn't enough. By eating constantly, from the time we wake up to the time we sleep, we prevent the activation of autophagy's cleansing pathways. Simply put, fasting cleanses the body of unhealthy or unnecessary cellular debris. This is the reason longer fasts were often called cleanses or detoxifications.

At the same time, fasting also improves growth hormone, which signals the production of some new snazzy cell parts, giving our bodies a complete renovation. Since it triggers both the breakdown of old cellular parts and the creation of new ones, fasting may be considered one of the most potent anti-aging methods in existence.

Autophagy also plays an important role in the prevention of Alzheimer's disease. Alzheimer's is characterized by the abnormal accumulation of amyloid beta (Aß) proteins in the brain, and it's believed that these accumulations eventually destroy the synaptic connections in the memory and cognition areas. Normally, clumps of Aß protein are removed by autophagy: the brain cell activates the autophagosome, the cell's internal garbage truck, which engulfs the Aß protein targeted for removal and excretes it, so it can be removed by the blood and recycled into other protein or turned into glucose, depending upon the body's needs. But in Alzheimer's disease, autophagy is impaired and the Aß protein remains inside the brain cell, where eventual buildup will result in the clinical syndromes of Alzheimer's disease.

Cancer is yet another disease that may be a result of disordered autophagy. We're learning that mTOR plays a role in cancer biology, and mTOR inhibitors have been approved by the Food and Drug Administration for the treatment of various cancers. Fasting's role in inhibiting mTOR, thereby stimulating autophagy, provides an interesting opportunity to prevent cancer's development. Indeed, some leading scientists, such as Dr. Thomas Seyfried, a professor of biology at Boston College, have proposed a yearly seven-day water-only fast for this very reason.

Fasting can limit growth of glucose-dependent tumors. Fasting can also target inflammation that contributes to the initiation and progression of tumors. We showed that fasting or calorie restriction could significantly reduce distal tumor invasion in our preclinical models of brain cancer.

CHAPTER 5: MORE ON KETOSIS AND FASTING

We are what we eat. It sounds like a simple sentence, straight forward, right? However, let's take it one step further and remember how we live. Chances are if you're reading this book you're trying to make a difference. Perhaps the target is weight loss, trying to lose the last ten pounds of fat. Maybe you're considering changing your diet and take preventive steps and put yourself on a healthier future health route.

Intermittent fasting and ketosis, also called IF and Keto, are possibly common words, or at least recognizable, when you first purchased this book. As comparison to fad diets, where you may see fast results that are difficult to sustain in the long run, both intermittent fasting and keto address the root systems of how you consume food and the choices you make with each meal. Intermittent fasting and keto are lifestyle improvements correctly applied, and long-term strategies for a safer, happier you.

The availability of information today means everything that we want to know about is at our disposal, or with one tap. Sometimes, the same convenience can leave you overwhelmed with details. How can you decode it all and decide whether intermittent fasting and keto are for you right? I did a deep dive into both approaches and explored the effects of both practices — implemented on their own and in combination — so that you can cut straight to the chase and continue your sporadic keto journey.

Approach this like you would any recipe before you set out to make adjustments–read the instructions from beginning to end first. Be sure you understand the science behind it all and not just how to do intermittent fasting and cook keto-friendly meals. Reading all of the introductory material will promote the transition to this new lifestyle and help you see through to completion the 4-Week Program.

Tempting as it may be to jump right through the 4-Week Plan and Recipes, bear in mind that the secret to success is a solid base. The words between this introduction and the recettes provide a good start for the bricks and mortar.

To the Naysayers be prepared.

Nowadays, everyone is an expert, ready to express their views whether they are accepted or not. Note that You alone are an authority on you. Now that you've read through the parts below, you'll know if intermittent keto is right for you. If you have any underlying health issues, of course, please consult a physician before making any adjustments to your diet and lifestyle.

KETOSIS

Carbohydrates, on the surface are a simple, often rapid, and inexpensive type of nutrition to power through every day. Think of all those grab-and-go snacks we associate with breakfast— granola bars, smoothies filled with fruit, muffins. We continue our mornings with carbs, and add them on as the day goes on.

Just because something is working doesn't mean that it's the most powerful way. To keep us healthy, the tissues and cells that make up our bodies need energy to perform daily functions. There are two primary sources that allow them to draw energy from the food we eat. Carbohydrates are one source of energy which converts to glucose. This is the latest pattern most of us are adopting. However, there is an alternative source, and a surprising one: fat. Yeah, the very thing you've been advised to restrict your entire life may just be the tool you need to get your metabolism started up. When our bodies metabolize food and break down fatty acids, organic compounds are released, called ketones. Ketones serve as the energy for keeping our muscles and cells going.

You've certainly used the word "metabolism" all your life but do you know exactly what it means? The term refers simply to the chemical reactions that are necessary to stay alive in any living organism. Of course, given the complexity of the human body our metabolism is anything but basic. Our bodies are at work, continuously. Even as we sleep, our cells construct and rebuild continuously. They have to draw the energy from within our bodies.

Glucose, which is what we break down carbs into after we eat them, is one way we can fuel our metabolism. Our latest Recommendations on Eating focus on carbs as the main energy source. Add in any extra sugars that we eat and the required daily portions of fruit, starchy vegetables, grains and plant-based protein sources (e.g., beans), and there is no lack of glucose in our bodies. The problem with this energy consumption model is that it leaves us running like hamsters on one of those axes. We burn energy but get nowhere, especially if we eat more carbs than our bodies can use in a day's work.

But I have omitted the other type of energy: fat. How exactly does that work? Is it possible that tapping into that alternate source of fuel would allow our bodies to more efficiently burn coal, with greater overall benefit to our health? We are back to the old notion of you being what you eat, but now think instead of the core principle when you burn what you eat. That is where ketosis comes in. Switching to a high-fat, moderate-protein low-carb diet helps the body to reach a ketosis state where you metabolize fat, causing a release of ketones to fuel our elaborate internal functions. After fatty acids are broken down the liver releases ketones.

Achieving a ketosis state is about equilibrium, but not the kind you're used to feeding. It turns out that our existing food pyramid, which instructs us to eat an disproportionate amount of energy-rich, carbohydrate-rich foods, is upside down. A more effective fueling strategy has fats at the top of your body, making up 60 to 80 percent of your diet; protein at 20 to 30 percent in the middle; and carbs (really disguised as glucose) at the bottom, making up only 5 to 10 percent of your daily diet.

KETO VS. PALEO

Evolution has a lot to tell us. The ability to cook our food using fire and energy alone is evidence that change can be a positive thing. A major difference occurred somewhere between our hunter-gatherer foraging lifestyle and the modern world today. Of course, we now have longer life spans but from a health perspective what about the quality of those extra years? The slow feeling that never seems to go away is maybe not just because you need to get extra sleep (although sleep is always good!).

When food is our bodies ' fuel, then it is fair to assume that what we consume influences our productivity. Put diesel in a vehicle that is built to run on petrol and the consequences are catastrophic. Is it possible that our bodies today are in a similar state, the result of the evolution of our systems to depend on carbs for energy as food became more readily available, rather than fat, as in our early days of existence? I know this sounds very much like championing a paleo diet, but although the ketogenic lifestyle looks similar, the basic philosophy of keto is very different. Keto is about developing a balance between what you consume and how your body works— that's why the emphasis is on clear macronutrient manipulation (fat, protein, starch, sugar, and fluid). Each calory is composed of unique macronutrients. Knowing why you are making these clear food decisions is critical to understanding the broader picture.

For example, fiber keeps us healthy, as it helps to move food through the digestive system. What goes in must come out and that cycle requires fiber. Protein helps to repair tissue, to generate enzymes and to create bones, muscles and skin. Fluids keep us hydrated— our cells, tissues, and organs can't function properly without them. The primary function of carbohydrates is to provide energy, but in order to do so, the body needs to turn it into glucose which has a ripple effect in the rest of the body. Carb intake is a delicate balance for people with diabetes due to its relation to the development of insulin from increased levels of blood sugar. Healthy fats promote cell growth, protect our lungs, help keep us warm and have the potential to provide energy, but only when small amounts of carbohydrates are eaten. I'll talk more about why and how that's going to happen soon.

CARBS VS. NET CARBS

For almost every food source, carbohydrates exist in some form. It is difficult and impractical to remove the carbohydrates entirely. We need to make some carbohydrates work. If we want to understand why some foods which fall into the restricted category on a keto diet are better choices than others, it is important to know this.

During the nutrient breakdown of a meal, fiber counts as carb. What's important to remember is that fiber doesn't affect our blood sugar significantly— a good thing, because it's an essential macronutrient that helps us digest the food properly. By subtracting the amount of fiber from the sum of carbs in an ingredient's nutritional count or finished recipe, you are left with what's called net carbs.

Think of your paycheck before (gross) income, and after (net). A bad comparison, maybe, as no one likes paying taxes but an important one in trying to grasp and track carbs versus net carbs. You put a certain amount of carbohydrates in your body, but they don't all affect your blood sugar.

It doesn't mean the all-grain pasta will go mad. While it's a better option than white-flour pasta, overall, your net carbs should be limited to 20 to 25 grams per day. Two ounces of uncooked whole grain pasta contain about 35 grams of carbohydrates and just 7 grams of total fiber. The two key things that people would ask you if you lack are probably pasta and bread. The best way to react to them is by sharing everything you can eat.

HOW Would IT TAKE TO KICK IN FOR KETOSIS?

Most people transition to ketosis within 1 to 3 days. This can take a full week for certain people, because all bodies are different. Factors influencing how easily you reach ketosis include your current body weight, diet and level of exercise.

To get into ketosis, the body has to burn first through its stock of glycogen (glucose). After the glycogens have been exhausted, it is time the body started breaking down those fatty acids. The liver gets the order to start excreting ketones over the next few days. This final part of the cycle is signalling you are in ketosis. The early stage is a mild ketosis, as the levels of ketone will be relatively small before you sustain ketosis for a steady time. You may officially calculate ketone levels but you may begin to note certain physiological changes indicating you are in ketosis, such as keto flu or keto breath. Symptoms aren't as serious or dramatic as symptoms sound, and the benefits of ketosis the outweigh the downside against your established goals during this phase-in time, but it's important to get to know the symptoms anyway.

FASTING INTERMITTENTLY: What does it mean?

Which is the first thing that comes to mind when you hear the sentence "I will fly today?" Let me guess — is it "hey I'm not going to starve to death"? With this common misunderstanding, you are not alone, so let's break it down and make it easier to swallow (pun very well intended!).

FASTING VS. STARVATION A deliberate decision is to fast. What separates fasting from hunger is that it's the choice not to feed intentionally. The amount of time you want to fast, and the intention of fasting (whether for religious purposes, weight loss or a detox) is not imposed upon you. Fasting occurs at will. Fasting is performed properly and can have beneficial effects on our overall wellbeing.

Starvation is unwillingly forced upon people by a series of conditions beyond their control, for starvation, hunger, and war are only a few explanations for such a disastrous situation. Starvation is a serious calorie deficit which can result in organ damage and eventually death. No one wants to starve to death.

This made complete sense when I was talking about not eating from this angle, so it was so much easier to wrap my mind around the notion. Indeed, I was cynical about fasting in the first place too. Once I knew that fasting and starvation varied, my first reaction to the thought of not eating was always "Why would anyone want to starve?"The fact is that someone who wants to run can only want not to eat for a predetermined period of time. Even peaceful protests which use fasting as a means to an end have a definite fasting aim.

WILL YOU FEEL HUNGRY FASTING WHILE?

Let's place the question in context for addressing that. The truth is, once a day we are all fast. We always eat our last meal a couple of hours before going to sleep, and I can't think of anything but breastfeeding newborns who feed the moment they wake. Even if you just average six hours of sleep a night, you probably already fast ten hours a day. Now let's add the sporadic concept to the mix. "Intermittent" means an uncontinuous event. When adding this to the concept of fasting, it means that you are prolonging the time that you are not eating between meals (the term "breakfast" means just that, breaking the quick).

Since our bodies are already used to fasting once a day, mind over matter is the bigger problem. Let's get back to the issue of feeling tired. The first week of your new fasting target can be an adjustment as you get used to the extended period of time.

It's quite likely that your body will start to feel hungry whatever time you're used to eating breakfast at the moment if it's before noon, but you'll change it within a few days.

In celebration of the shift you're about to make, consider moving back your first meal of the day for a week per day by thirty minutes before you launch the 4-Week Program.

WHY SHOULD YOU CHOOSE INTERMITTENT FASTING?

Now that we've explained what fasting actually means and you know it's a deliberate decision not to eat for a while, you might still ask, why bother? The primary reason intermittent fasting (commonly known as IF) took the world of diet by storm is its potential to encourage weight loss. Metabolism is also graded as one of human body functions. Metabolism generally requires two basic reactions: catabolism and anabolism.

Catabolism is the aspect of the metabolism by which our bodies break down the food we eat. Complex molecules are broken down into smaller units during catabolism which release energy. Instead anabolism uses the energy to start the process of restoring and repairing our bodies, forming new cells and holding tissues. Practically speaking, catabolism and anabolism occur at the same time, but the pace they occur at is different. A conventional food routine, where we spend most of our day eating, means that our bodies have less energy to spend in the second, or anabolic, metabolism level. It's perhaps a little complicated, since the processes are interdependent, but note that the levels they occur at vary. The key lesson here is that fasting in the metabolic processes over an elongated time allows over optimum efficiency.

The impressive side-effect of fasting is a revival in mental acuity, even for an intermittent time as illustrated in this novel. Numerous studies show that fasting, contrary to common opinion, can make you more alert and concentrated, not exhausted or light-headed.

Some point to nature and our need to survive as a species: long before food survival was possible, there was still a need for mental knowledge so that we could live from day to day, no matter how plentiful food supplies may have been.

Scientific evidence points to neurogenesis, the growth and development of nerve tissue in the brain, which kicks into high gear during fasting times.

All paths lead to one incredibly significant conclusion when it comes to fasting: giving the body time to do some of the required work behind the scenes. The longer you prolong the period between consuming one day's last meal and consuming the next day's first meal, the more time the body requires to concentrate on cellular regeneration and tissue repair at all stages.

When Fasting Is Liquids Allowed?

There is one more important detail on intermittent fasting to remember. Unlike religious fasting, which usually limits fast intake of either food or liquid, IF allows you to drink other liquids. Technically speaking, a fast breaks the moment you eat something with calories. Looking at it for its weight-loss advantages through the prism by using intermittent fasting means we can apply various guidelines.

To order to replenish vitamins and minerals and control sodium levels, bone broth is recommended. Coffee and tea are required, ideally without added milk or cream and with no sweeteners at all. There are two think tanks to add milk to your coffee or tea. Given that making bulletproof coffee is just a high-fat addition, such as coconut oil or butter, many keto proponents think its perfect, because it does not interfere with ketosis. It's assumed that adding MCT (medium-chain triglyceride) oil raises energy levels and also makes you feel sated. Purists stick with plain tea or coffee. You will do for you what works best, so you don't get kicked out of ketosis.

Don't forget about water, since staying well hydrated is important for any healthy lifestyle choices. Caffeine can be especially depleting so make sure your coffee consumption is always balanced with water intake.

THE POWER OF INTERMITTENT FASTING & KETO COMBINED
The benefits of intermittent fasting and adherence to a keto diet should be apparent by now. What you might not have pieced together is the relation between the two. The cycle of breaking down fatty acids to create ketones for fuel when you're in ketosis is basically what the body does to keep going while you're fasting. How does combining the two mean, and why bother mixing certain behaviors and eating ways?

Fasting for one to two days has a major impact of consuming a conventional diet based on carb. After the initial energy burning step of glucose (that is, carbohydrates), the body turns naturally to burning fat as fuel.

You see where I'm at, right? When it takes the body twenty-four to forty-eight hours to turn to burning fat for food, consider the consequences of mixing intermittent keto-fasting. To maintain a constant ketosis state means your body already burns fat for fuel. That means the longer you spend in a fasting state, the longer you burn the fat. Intermittent fasting combined with keto makes the weight-loss effects of fasting more effective and also leads to more weight loss than conventional diets. The extended time between the last and the first meals of the day ensures the body has extra fat-burning capability.

Ketosis is sometimes used in body building, because it is a healthy way to shed fat without muscle loss. Weight loss is only effective when the weight is right and we all need muscle mass to stay healthy.

HOW THAT WORK IT?

Turning to keto diet is a huge shift in lifestyle. That is why it is best to ease into this program's intermittent fasting aspect. Let your body adjust to a new way of eating, adapt to fat burning for food, and deal with any potential side effects (remember that keto flu is a possibility) before integrating intermittent fasting into your eating routine, or in this case, your extended eating time. Note that intermittent fasting is not implemented in the 4-Week Schedule until Week 2.

You'll want to take care of the meal times during the phase-in process. Your last meal of the day will be no later than 6 p.m., even before you implement the intermittent-fasting portion of the schedule. It should make fasting easier for you, and help prevent snacking. One of the keto results is that it teaches your body— and your brain, let's face it — to eat only when you're hungry. With the passage of time, cravings stop. They sometimes equate cravings with hunger because it is a learned action to have cravings, when hunger is a physiological demand to refill our energy reserves.

TIMING YOUR FASTING Cycle This is a little versatile how you want to implement your intermittent-fasting time. Do you prefer to dive first into the head of the pool, or do you first dip your toes? Knowing that your temperament will help you find out which routine is best for you. In talking to my editor while writing this novel, I discovered that it wasn't her that was appealing to me.

I don't like getting in a rut and breakfast is one of my favorite meals of the day, so for me, having an alternative routine that allows me to eat breakfast and abstain from dinner just about every other day, and doing the opposite on the other days (fasting through breakfast and eating dinner), is preferable. My writer, Marisa, likes consistency, something that I think a lot of people would like to do as well— to go on auto-pilot and fly every day at the same time. I can see how one or the other can work into other behaviors and mindsets, and that's why two schedules are to be chosen. They let you tailor the Intermittent Keto Program to suit your lifestyle best.

BEFORE YOU GET STARTED Looking at the big picture of every situation is crucial to long term success. This is especially true for significant changes in diet and lifestyle. Intermittent keto throws everything you thought you learned about food, when to eat, and when to eat it out of the window. It's not a leap-out-looking kind of decision, so it's crucial to get acquainted with what to expect, how to tackle possible obstacles, and how to reorganize your life in a way that helps you to meet your goals before you start.

DEFINE YOUR GOALS Why were you opting to try intermittent keto? Is that justified for health? Missing weight? Looking to just feel better and increase your energy levels? Is this supposed to be a short-term detox or are you trying to make lifestyle changes for the long term? When do you intend to follow up on your macronutrients? Would you intend on checking for ketones to make sure you have entered a ketosis state? You are vegetarian, or you are vegan?

Before you start, all of these are important questions to ask so you can remain focused on achieving your objective. Evidence shows that intermittent fasting will offer significant benefits in the long term. The jury is still out on the benefits of adopting a keto diet indefinitely, or any possible risks. The Plan's rigidity often determines how long people stick to it.

Also, the way you eat at the moment is a huge concern when doing keto, so you should realize how huge a shift or challenge that could pose. Keto is a macronutrient-wise, fat-focused diet but protein plays an significant role. Too little protein, during ketosis, can cause muscle failure. Too much from ketosis will get you kicked. It's a compromise, and although keto isn't a high-protein diet, the default protein is always meat because the plant-based protein alternatives usually reported are too high in carbs relative to their fiber and protein ratio, specifically beans, like tofu (made from soybeans).

This doesn't mean you can't stay vegetarian on keto, particularly if you are a vegetarian ovo-lacto (okay with consuming eggs and dairy). Examples of non-meat protein which are not legumes include eggs, nuts, beans, and cheese. This book's recipes are geared towards an omnivorous diet. Meat is a feature of several of the recettes. You will need to tailor your meal plan, supplementing it with outside source recipes. The majority of the information found in this book will be highly useful, and this will also extend to vegans. It's not difficult if you choose to try intermittent keto with a vegan diet, but it does take much more careful preparation to make sure you don't push yourself out of ketosis by selecting protein sources too high in carbs. Some of the recipes in this book would need to be tailored to your dietary needs, too.

Ketosis testing can be performed in three ways: urine test strips; a blood ketone test (with a meter similar to the blood glucose level test); and a breath test (different from keto breath, discussed separately). Urine tests are considered the least reliable, but they are the least costly, the most accurate being blood meters. As you may have guessed, they are also the most expensive.

The real question is to check yourself for ketones? If your aim is to lose weight, and the pounds drop, plus you're feeling good (well rested and energetic) after the first few weeks, ketosis testing could be a moot point. If it comes to counting numbers, the more critical factor is tracking what you consume.

Macronutrients vs. Calories: What are you relying on?

Tracking your macronutrients is different from mere calorie counting. With keto, the focus is on controlling the amount of fat, protein and carbohydrates you consume— all macronutrients have a similar calorie count: 1 gram of fat= 9 calories, 1 gram of protein= 4 calories, 1 gram of carbohydrate= 4 calories. Indeed, it is just closer analysis of any calorie consumed. A baseline metabolic rate, also referred to as BMR, is also required to decide how many calories you will consume for weight maintenance and weight loss (another explanation why it's important to identify your goals).

Both these macronutrients play a crucial role both in your overall health and in maintaining and remaining in ketosis, but carbohydrates are the one that gets the most attention on keto as they result in glucose during digestion, which is the source of energy that you are trying to keep your body away from using. Some research indicates the average amount of total carbs that one can eat on keto per day is 50 grams or less— which results in 20 to 35 net carbs per day, depending on the fiber content. The lower you can get the net carbs down, the quicker your body goes into ketosis and the easier it is going to be to stay there.

Keep in mind that we're recommending 20 grams of net carbs a day, depending on how many calories you need to eat based on your BMR, the fat and protein grams are variables. The recommended daily average for women for weight maintenance ranges between 1,600 and 2,000 calories, depending on activity level (from sedentary to active). Adhering to a daily diet of consuming 160 grams of fat + 70 grams of protein + 20 grams of carbohydrates parallels 1,800 calories of eating— the optimal number for moderately active women (walking 1.5 to 3 miles a day) according to the USDA for weight maintenance. If you have a sedentary lifestyle — defined as exercising from usual daily activities such as cleaning and walking short distances only — you would like to see 130 grams of fat + 60 grams of protein + 20 grams of carbohydrates jump-start weight loss (1500 calories). There are plenty of online calculators to calculate your BMR and overall calorie goal, and to calculate the right fat / protein ratio while maintaining net carbs at 20 grams per day.

Speaking of calculators and tracking numbers, you may find it helpful to create from the recipes in this book a tracking system for your macronutrients to help you customize your own specific menu.

It can be as simple as writing it down and doing the calculations in a notebook, but it may be more time consuming. There's no lack of software for your phone to make monitoring macronutrients simple too.

THE PHYSICAL SIDE EFFECTS OF KETO Unlike diet plans that merely limit the weight loss foods you consume, keto goes deeper. Ketosis is about changing how you eat and how your body turns what you eat into energy. The ketosis cycle changes the balance from burning glucose (remember, carbs), to burning fat for fuel instead. This comes with potential side effects while the body is adapting to a new way of functioning. It is also why the phases of the 4-Week Program after week two of intermittent fasting, and not from the get-go. It's crucial that you give yourself time to adjust properly, both physically and mentally. The keto flu and keto breath are two physical changes you may encounter when you transition to a keto diet.

KETO FLU

Keto flu, also referred to as carb flu, can last from a few days to several weeks anywhere. With the body weaning itself from consuming glucose for energy, metabolic changes may result in increased feelings of lethargy, irritability, muscle soreness, lightheadedness or brain fog, changes in bowel movements, nausea, stomach discomfort, and difficulty concentrating and concentration. I know, that sounds horrible, and probably vaguely familiar. Indeed, all these are typical flu symptoms, and hence the name.

The good news is that the body learns this is a brief process and it doesn't impact everybody. Factors that cause these symptoms include an excess of electrolytes (sodium, potassium, magnesium and calcium) and elimination of sugar from the substantially reduced intake of carbohydrates. Expecting these potential symptoms means that, should it arise, you should be prepared to relieve them and reduce the duration of keto flu.

The amount of highly processed foods you eat is directly influencing the sodium levels. To be specific, all we consume is a processed food technically; the word means "a set of steps taken to achieve a particular goal." Only cooking from scratch at home involves the act of processing food. Nevertheless, with regard to our modern society, where ready-to-eat foods are available at any turn of the supermarket, these highly refined products continue to contain exorbitant amounts of secret salt (sodium is both a preservative and a taste enhancer).

This is most effective to stick to a keto diet when you do the actual cooking, so you can monitor the number of carbohydrates and the amount of sugar in a bowl. Home cooking appears to be less refined, which may lead to lower sodium, too. It's fast, natural ways to raise your sodium levels by increasing the amount of salt in your food and drinking a homemade stock such as the bone broth.

Certain foods for focusing on during your keto phase-in time are listed below. To help keep the electrolytes in order, they are naturally high in magnesium, potassium and calcium.

Magnesium (helps with muscle soreness and leg cramps) Avocados, broccoli, pork, kale, almonds, pumpkin seeds, spinach Potassium (helps with muscle soreness, hydration) Asparagus, avocados, Brussels sprouts, salmon, tomatoes, leafy vegetables Calcium (especially essential if you were a big pre-keto milk drinker) Almonds, bok choy, broccoli, cabbage, collard greens, spinach, sardines, sesame and chia see It can be as easy as exchanging your morning muffin for a hard-boiled or scrambled egg, skipping the bun and covering your burger in lettuce (often called protein-style when ordering), or switching out spaghetti for zoodles. This way it would feel more like a normal step of eating less carbs as you dive into the program than a sudden right turn in your diet.

KETO BREATH Let's cut here for chase. Bad breath stinks, literally, but when you turn to keto it is something you should be bracing yourself for. There are 2 ideas as to why this is happening.

When the body enters ketosis and begins releasing ketones (a by-product of burning fat for fuel), one of the released ketones is acetone (yes, the same solvent used in nail polish remover and paint thinners). During the body's effort to finish the biochemical cycle of breaking down certain fatty acids, acetone is excreted by urine and through your breath. It can lead to unpleasant breath-smelling.

Protein can also be a factor in helping to breathe keto. Note, high fat, moderate protein and low carb are the macronutrient targets. People also believe high protein fat is interchangeable. Which isn't real anyway. Fat and protein are digested differently by the body. When breaking down protein, our bodies generate ammonia, and typically release it during urine production. Eating more protein than you need results in residual indigestible levels in your digestive system, where it ferments, creating ammonia, which is then released through your intake.

The positive is that the body is in ketosis, keto breath is a clear sign. How long the odor lasts can vary depending on how well the body adapts to ketosis. Some reports say it lasts from a week to just under a month, everywhere. A deeper dive into the keto message boards and chat groups reveals that it can last for months, although some people say that they never encounter. Any strategies to stop or minimize keto breath should always be prepared with sugar-free gum, reduce your protein intake, ensure that you adhere to a healthy dental routine (brushing and flossing), and follow the advice provided earlier on lowering your carbohydrate intake slowly until you jump full steam into the 4-Week Program.

SLEEP & EXERCISE A healthy lifestyle requires ample sleep and moderate exercise. When identifying your priorities and finding out how the two blend into your everyday life, the same advice should be considered. When you integrate intermittent fasting into your strategy, those sleeping hours are even more important because they are part of your time to run. Hold snacking impulses at bay late at night, by tucking in at a decent time.

Weight training is a big focus among keto enthusiasts and when you're in maintenance mode, it's definitely necessary. Cardio workouts offer the greatest fat-burning boost when it comes to weight loss. When you have ongoing health problems, make sure to contact your doctor before making any big changes.

TALK WITH YOUR FRIENDS & FAMILY Mention the word "diet" and you'll find that most people have strong opinions about other diet plans that increase in severity. Everybody has the right to their thoughts and often sharing common experiences is beneficial when you're looking for inspiration or motivation. What's not helpful is when people think, "You look fine the way you are" or "I could never give up carbs" or, worse, "You're going to starve yourself?!"Every ship needs a helmsman so make yourself your body's helmsman. There will be friends and family to help you on this journey so motivate them with the knowledge to do so. If you are confident thinking about it, let them know why you're making the move. At the very least clarify the ideas behind why for certain people intermittent fasting and keto work very well. People are still simply puzzled about what they don't know, and don't take the time to try answers. If they want to look further into the diet, you can even send them a copy of this book! You never know if you're going to inspire someone to try sporadic keto too, and then you're going to have a friend to keep track of success, set goals and keep each other inspired.

Sharing the decision to go on keto is also a safe way to avoid turning up at a dinner party with a friend and finding that they only serve pasta. Under such a situation, you will be volunteering to put in a meal to share that is also keto-friendly to enjoy. This way it relieves any burden that your host may have on cooking for you, plus it highlights some of the great foods you can eat on keto!

There'll be those who believe they know better, or insist that stealing here and there is okay. Perhaps that works with other diets but by eating too many carbohydrates you can quickly knock yourself out of ketosis. Make yourself a strong friend, and don't be afraid to say no thank you. People who care for you will value your hard work in creating a healthy lifestyle for themselves, and will not seek to tempt you.

Obviously, when making arrangements, you want to bear in mind your intermittent fasting schedule too. Late-night dinners don't always get in the way of the schedule, so you should get together for drinks and keep your order to have a regular seltzer with a lime wedge, or better yet meet for a coffee after dinner. The 4-Week Plan was designed to give you a break from intermittent Sunday morning fasting, keeping in mind that gathering with friends is a common time and brunch is very easy to adhere to on the keto diet.

STAYING IN KETOSIS & WHAT HAPPENS IF YOU FALL OUT OF IT

When you reach ketosis, it's up to you for how long you want to stick to it after you finish the 4-Week Program. Is your target just to drop a size dress? A month could be all you need. Have you been trying to get rid of sugar or raising the average consumption of carb? Perhaps it could take a little longer to help set long-term eating habits even if you plan to increase the overall carb count above the 20 grams per day allotted in the 4-Week Program. Technically something less than 50 grams of carbohydrates (in general, not net carbs) helps push your body into fat-burning mode, so even a slight increase in carbs will give a mild ketosis advantage, even though you may get back some of the pounds you initially lost.

Be prepared for curves and potential pitfalls to understand. When you eat too much fat, too many sugars or don't get enough exercise, it's possible to force the body out of ketosis. A simple error, or simply a craving like consuming a sweet potato, will bring you back in the state of glucose-burning.

When keto sounds strict, it's because it is. Going into ketosis and sustaining it is a commitment-that's why we talked early on about setting your goals. Though after all the hard work you put in it could seem terrible or frustrating, don't beat yourself up. Reflect on your potential objectives, and get back to ketosis. Should not prolong the cheat, saying, "Ah, well, the harm is done." Instead, fasting after a day of cheat is one way to get back on track, keeping in mind that you will have to burn through the glucose first again.

Journaling is a perfect way to track more than just calories, in general. Start tracking how you feel mentally, and what your mental attitude is— a simple number rating system lets you understand whether you're making improvements, keeping the status quo, or sliding along with your objectives. Detailed notes could help recognize more direct reasons for your cheat day to help you prepare better in the future. Yes, you may want to pad in cheat days so you can foresee them, rather than beating yourself up for getting them. If you know the wedding of your best friend is coming up and you're going to want to engage in the celebrations 100 percent, including all the food and drink served, prepare for that. While you can not simply turn a switch to get back into ketosis, you should know what to expect and potentially get back on track faster than the first time. Also worth noting is that you don't have to rely on too many cheat days. That goes back to describing your goals once again.

KNOW WHAT FOODS TO ENJOY & WHAT FOODS TO AVOID

KETO CHEAT SHEET

Eat: Puréed cauliflower

Avoid: Mashed potatoes

Eat: Cauliflower rice, shirataki rice

Avoid: Rice, couscous

Eat: Zoodles, spaghetti squash and shirataki noodles

Avoid: Pasta

Eat: Heavy cream and cheeses (mozzarella, cheddar)

Avoid: Milk

Eat: Low-carb tortillas and keto bread

Avoid: Bread, wraps, tortillas

Eat: Zucchini fries

Avoid: French fries and sweet potato fries

Eat: Use almond flour, unsweetened coconut flakes and pork cracklings

Avoid: Bread crumbs

Eat: Meat, poultry, seafood, eggs

Avoid: Beans, tofu

Eat: Stevia, monk fruit

Avoid: Sweeteners (honey, maple syrup, sugar)

Eat: Olive oil, coconut oil, avocado oil, butter, ghee, sesame oil (in small quantities)

Avoid: Sunflower, grapeseed, canola, peanut, safflower oils, margarine, vegetable shortening

Eat: Water (key for staying hydrated), coffee, tea

Avoid: Sugary drinks (soda, juices), alcohol

Eat: Berries; use lemons and limes for flavor

Avoid: Sweet citrus (oranges, grapefruit, clementines), tropical fruits (bananas, mango, pineapple), all dried fruits

Eat: Parmesan Crisps

Avoid: Chips and sweet/salty snacks

THE KETO KITCHEN It's crucial to ensure that your pantry aligns with your new eating goals up to the intermittent keto launch. Those new priorities may also be at odds with the majority of your household members, whether they are family members or roommates. If so, it may not be possible to remove all the carb-laden foods, sugary snacks and refined foods. In that case, it will be a self-control exercise for you, particularly within the first week or two, when cravings can be difficult to handle. Don't worry. You can always assert a kitchen area, and set up a keto-friendly area to make it easier to adhere to the program. And by all means, if you live alone, or if your partner / family does this with you, go full throttle and use a modern, out-with - the-old approach. Instead of discarding unwanted items, donate them to a local grocery store (check the expiration dates first), or send them to your neighbours.

When you have a clean slate, it's time to begin to fill the pantry with all the food you might enjoy. Below are some of the key items to add to your first shopping list.

Fermented products (make sure the vegetables are lacto-fermented): pickles, kimchi, sauerkraut, plain full-fat yogurt Oils: avocado oil, extra virgin olive oil, cold-pressed or virgin coconut oil, ghee, MCT oil Nuts and seeds (and flours made from them): almonds, walnuts, macadamia nuts, brazilian nuts, pecans, chia seeds, pumpkin seeds, sunflower seeds, sesame seeds, almond flour or meal, coconut flour Canned flour

A WORD ABOUT BAKING POWDER & OTHER INGREDIENTS

One look at the ingredients and you'll find that the commercial baking powder contains cornstarch. In reality it's even in most homemade recipes. Baking powder is typically made with a mixture of baking soda, tartar cream, and cornstarch. Some keto people will warn you that cornstarch is completely prohibited, since it's a grain and you shouldn't eat any grains on keto. It is important to note, however, that you shouldn't eat grains until you decide on a decision about baking powder. The main explanation for this is that grains are high on starch, and keto is low-carb diet. The truth is, the amount of cornstarch in baking powder is so small when opposed to how much you actually use in a recipe that it barely registers. If, for health reasons, you're grain free, that's a perfect excuse to make your own baking powder or look for a brand without any cornstarch. I have yet to find one that exists, but the printing of this book will change that. All of the recipes were checked in this book using store-bought baking powder. Results aren't assured using a homemade version without cornstarch.

Throughout the healing process most bacon has added sugar, even bacon from small, artisanal farms. While the actual amount of sugar in the finished product is small, if you have trouble balancing your carb count you may want to look for a brand that has no added sugar.

The ketchups are not all made together. Most are simply filled with sugar. Purchase an unsweetened brand such as Primal Kitchen for dipping and make the BBQ sauce for sure.

Many keto fans swear by MCT oil. It is not coconut oil but rather a coconut by-product. MCT stands for triglycerides in the medium chain. Among the health benefits that it is said to deliver is that it keeps you satiated (feeling full), offers a rapid boost in energy and promotes a strong immune system. The maximum sensation it gives may be why some people believe it helps to lose weight, stopping you from over-eating or snacking.

WEEKLY GROCERY SHOPPING When it comes to processing, all herbs are given a green light — great news because they are simple flavor boosters for every meal. For vegetables the general rule of thumb is that you should stick to those that grow above ground. That means keeping clear of root vegetables and tubers (think carrots, parsnips, beets, onions, and standard and sweet potatoes), as they're higher in carbohydrates than starchy vegetables. Many vegetables above level, too, are high-carb, like winter squash, potato, corn, and peas.

You can also consume the rainbow, so don't panic-cool, leafy greens (kale, spinach), broccoli, cauliflower, zucchini (zoodles!), radishes, cucumbers, garlic, asparagus, mushrooms, and eggplant all enter the list for keto meals.

Fruit lovers can find keto difficult, as most fruits are too high in natural sugars and therefore off-limits, particularly dried fruits—which have higher sugar levels. Basically, the options are berries (because they're mainly fibre), lemon, and limes. All other citrus fruits are extremely rich in natural sugar. Yet can you know what? If in some dishes you love an orange essence, you can use orange zest to add colour without having any of the carbs!

You might feel weighted down by all the things you can't eat at this stage. That's a natural feeling, and while it's a fact if you're dedicated to keto, I just tend to concentrate on the food you can eat, snap a picture of the Keto Cheat Sheet here and you'll always have a fast point of reference when in doubt.

Critical Cooking Equipment Veteran cooks currently have a well stocked kitchen. If you just start, you will quickly realize that cooking your own food improves your ability to adhere to a keto diet. I try to stay away from devices that only serve one reason but my spiralizer and avocado slicer are exceptions to that law. Homemade zoodles are a breeze to make with my handheld spiralizer, which is sold in the kitchen section of the hardware store for under $20.

The avocados are a favorite of keto fans. Pitting avocados also leads to more visits to the emergency room than you would expect, and can even cause nerve damage. This happened to a close friend of mine, who is a chef with experience. Now she owns an avocado slicer.

As for skillets, if you can buy only one set of pans, I consider nonstick to be perfect. While in your current diet you can consume considerably more fat, non-stick skillets are perfect for making eggs and pancakes (check out the Blueberry Almond Pancakes here).

Here is a list of cooking devices and equipment that you can find helpful when preparing meals:

8-inch skillet

Spiralizer

10-inch skillet

Digital kitchen scale

Bento box for packing lunches

Avocado slicer

Tongs and spatula

Silicon candy molds (for making fat bombs)

Variety of saucepans (ranging from two quarts to four quarts, if space and budget permit)

Chef's knife and paring knife

Mason jars (for preparing and transporting chia puddings)

Cutting boardsBlender

Chef's knife and paring knife

Food processor (optional, but especially helpful to grind your own nut flours)

WHEN TO STOP & HOW TO STOP

Keto is strict on what you can eat, and can't. Throw in extended fasting, and further limit your eating time. It is a good time to think about how long you can live on the keto and start your intermittent fasting before you dive into your 4-Week Program. There is actually not enough evidence to conclude from a health perspective regarding the long-term efficacy of keto, but the fact is that you are struggling against the innate instinct of your body to run on glucose itself. Even though we have developed under the idea of fat for heat, times have changed and our bodies have changed along with that — for better or for worse.

Although there is a lack of studies offering clear hypotheses about how the keto diet functions (apart from those relevant to specific medical issues), several people lean to using keto many times a year for a prolonged period of time— anywhere from a few weeks to a few months — taking a break in between while always being mindful of total carb intake.

Intermittent fasts are another matter. I know someone who has been fasting for a few years now, intermittently. Her strategy is different from the program outlined here, and she's not on keto, so her background is different, but she has been very effective and manageable in managing intermittent fasting. She's also one of the biggest foodies and cooks I know and her style hasn't been cramped by intermittent fasting a bit. In reality quite the reverse. As they leave their feeling refreshed and centered, she looks forward to her fast days. I recommend you do some work to figure out the right strategy and plan for yourself, if you want to step away from the keto diet and stick with intermittent fasting.

You have to do so meaningfully and methodically when you believe you have reached the end of your keto journey, or just want to stop for a time beyond a cheat. Know the body has taken time to adapt to ketosis. The same goes with a diet that has more sugars, turning the switch back to fat consuming glucose. That applies even though the goal is to remain on a diet that is lower in carb than you eat until keto begins.

If you decide to turn off keto, points to bear in mind are: take it slowly, add more carbs at a time.

Expect to gain some weight. The sum of the keto depends on how long you have been on. The initial weeks of keto weight loss appears to be water weight. The weight gain will be lower if you've been on keto for a while, because you're not overindulging in carbohydrates and sugar.

Familiarize yourself with balanced portion sizes once again, changing the fat and protein content accordingly.

CONCLUSION

Fasting — where you limit calorie consumption for a prolonged period of time — appears to bring some very surprising health benefits with it. These include weight loss, improvements to the diabetes and heart disease risk factors, and longer life.

Researchers have sought to get to the bottom of why fasting has long been related to longevity. Labor mice and monkeys that are swift in laboratory studies continue to live longer than their regularly fed peers.

Research reveals that calorie restriction flips on genes that tell cells to conserve food. The cells enter a survival or "famine mode," where they are substantially more resistant to disease or cell stress. They also begin a cycle known as autophagy, where the body begins cleaning up the old, discarded, and unneeded cellular material, and repairing and recycling damaged parts.

In one test, mice that fasted for 24 hours showed high autophagosomal numbers, the signs that autophagy works. Now we need to be careful to connect this directly to humans, since the metabolism of the mouse is much faster than ours. Although autophagy is very difficult to test outside of a laboratory setting, many experts agree that after 18-20 hours of fasting, the autophagy cycle begins in humans, with maximum benefits occurring once the 48–72 hour mark has been reached. If this sounds overwhelming, bear in mind that doing intermittent fasts will still give you benefits, but occasionally (a few times a year depending on your personal risk factors) you can recommend taking a longer time to enable autophagy entirely and do some spring cleaning for your cells. You will, of course, also consult your doctor before you embark on any fasting regimen.

Stimulating autophagy does many things: it cleans out old, unwanted cellular materials and proteins, and it also increases growth hormone development, which regenerates fresh cellular material and speeds up cell regeneration. When the body has had an infection recently, autophagy can be able to kill the persistent bacteria or viruses.

Autophagy is not only related to rising survival, it helps researchers understand degenerative diseases like Parkinson's and Alzheimer's better. If autophagy does not occur regularly, a variety of cellular material is accumulated by the body, including proteins that appear in significant quantities in Alzheimer's, Parkinson's, and even cancer: amyloid beta or Tau protein. Scientists suggest that repeated autophagy bouts may clear the brains of these excess proteins, thereby preventing the development of these diseases.

Where to get autophagy?

Although drug makers are working to develop a prescription panacea to induce autophagy, and some blogs on diet and fitness say that some supplements can activate autophagy, there is only one known way to trigger it: by fasting. Deprivation of nutrients causes autophagy.

Autophagy signaling in the body involves two main pathways when the nutrients of the body become depleted: mTOR, or rapamycin mammalian target, regulates nutrients which affect cell development, protein synthesis, and anabolism. It's related to insulin receptor activation and the development of new tissue.

AMPK or AMP-activated protein kinase helps preserve an energy homeostasis and activate the mechanisms of the body's fuel backup.

MTOR and AMPK are both attuned to the nutrient content of your body. These two pathways help your body determine whether to activate a response to growth — mTor— or go into autophagy — AMPK.

Autophagy acts with two main hormones: glucagon and insulin in concert too. People with diabetes or hypoglycemia have or are excessively responsive to insulin and have difficulty controlling. As insulin rises, glucagon descends, and vice versa. You drop insulin when you are heavy, and increase glucagon, which stimulates autophagy.

But, it's not that simple: You need low liver glycogen to cause autophagy, which is normally only done after around 14–16 hours of fasting, but is much more likely to happen after 24 hours, so it's a serious commitment.

Given these awesome advantages, the fasting level needed to enable autophagy is not for everyone. Some people feel low-energy, moody and during these fasts they have trouble sleeping. Strive for consistency and check with the healthcare providers at all times.

www.ingramcontent.com/pod-product-compliance
Lightning Source LLC
Chambersburg PA
CBHW081733250726
48657CB00010B/3249